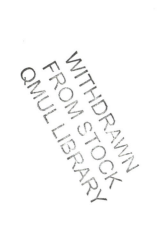

Color Atlas of

MINOR
ORAL SURGERY

Karl R Koerner
DDS, MS, FAGD, FICD

President, Institute for Applied Dental Learning,
Lecturer and Clinician on Oral Surgery,
Private Practice in Logan and Salt Lake City, Utah

Lloyd V Tilt
DDS, MS

Vice President, Institute for Applied Dental Learning,
Lecturer and Clinician on Periodontics,
Private Practice in Ogden, Utah

Kenneth R Johnson
DMD, MAGD

Private Practice, Corvalis, Oregon

N Mosby-Wolfe

London Baltimore Bogotá Boston Buenos Aires Caracas Carlsbad, CA Chicago Madrid Mexico City Milan Naples, FL New York Philadelphia St. Louis Sydney Tokyo Toronto Wiesbaden

Exclusive distribution worldwide,
except Spain:

ℕ Mosby-Wolfe

Times Mirror International Publishers Ltd.

Lynton House
7-12 Tavistock Square
LONDON - WC1H 9LB
England

ISBN: 0.7234.2038.6

A CIP catalogue record for this book is available from the British Library

© Espaxs, S.A. Publicaciones Médicas, 1994
Rosselló, 132
08036 - Barcelona
(Spain)

Printed in Spain

PREFACE

Oral surgery is a basic need of mankind. At its most fundamental level, it involves the removal of painful and diseased teeth and the establishment of drainage to prevent the spread of infection. Beyond this point we find a progression of procedures that ranges from those that support and enhance exodontia to others that have become quite specialized and sophisticated, even on the cutting edge of modern technology.

Regardless of patient need or the training and experience of the dental surgeon, there is a certain unchanging commonality within oral surgery; namely, the principles by which these procedures should be performed. Therefore, this book addresses the use of universal surgical principles that must be understood and practiced by anyone, anywhere who was earned the title of "dentist". It emphasizes treatment that is more traditional than avant-garde, i.e., exodontia, surgical extractions, impaction surgery, alveoplasty, lesion excision, apicoectomies, and alveolar ridge preservation with localized grafting. However, it digresses to include some operations that complement other dental disciplines such as surgical crown lengthening, free gingival grafts, frenectomies, and bracketing unerupted teeth for orthodontics.

This publication is an educational tool utilizing teaching methods that will simplify and enhance learning. They include outlines, written descriptions, lists and tables, flowcharts, line drawings, and hundreds of color plates. Multiple examples are presented, many with sequencing of surgical cases. It covers not only surgical technique, but case selection commensurate with operator ability, the prevention and treatment of complications, and patient management. It promotes a positive, "can do" attitude for generalists. It is geared to the generalist, yet recognizes the need for referral to specialist colleagues when they are available. The authors hope this book will further the accumulation and advancement of knowledge in this somewhat limited but vitally important area of human health.

Karl R. Koerner, DDS

NOTICE

Dentistry is an ever-changing science. As new research and clinical experience broaden our knowledge, changes in treatment are required. The editors and the publisher of this work have made every effort to ensure that the procedures herein are accurate and in accord with the standards accepted at the time of publication.

CONTENTS

Chapter 1

The Common Elements of Minor Oral Surgery

INTRODUCTION

Virtually all minor oral surgery procedures can be reduced to their more fundamental components, or *elements*. Each operation requires that the dentist be familiar with at least one, and often several, of those basic elements. Even though within the profession surgical procedures are often grouped by discipline into general oral surgery, endodontics, or periodontics, the surgical principles and other characteristics of which they are composed remain the same.

The general dentist must become competent with each of these elements. Once this expertise is attained, it is not difficult to perform a wide range of different yet related surgical procedures in the dental office. The five common elements consist of operations such as those listed in Table 1.

1

Table 1-1. Common Elements of Surgery

Soft Tissue Excision
- gingivoplasty
- gingivectomy
- small lesion removal
- graft donor site excision

Full-Thickness Mucoperiosteal Flap
- with flap reapposed
- with repositioning (apically, coronally)

Partial-Thickness Flap
- tissue excision (as with an autogenous free graft recipient bed)
- tissue repositioning (as with a pedicle graft)

Bone Excision
- removal for access
- removal to establish physiologic contours

Tooth Manipulation
- section cut
- apicoectomy
- purchase point
- hemisection
- root amputation
- recontouring

DISCUSSION OF EACH COMMON ELEMENT

Soft Tissue Excision

Soft tissue—attached gingiva, alveolar mucosa, developmental tissue, or pathologic growths—frequently needs to be excised from the mouth. Two examples of attached gingiva procedures are the gingivoplasty and gingivectomy. In either alveolar or attached mucosa, there could also be a need for biopsy to include small lesion removal. The excision of a distal wedge posterior to a lower second molar might involve both attached and unattached tissue. Follicles and granulomatous lesions are other types of soft tissue requiring excision. *See Figs. 1-1 through 1-3.*

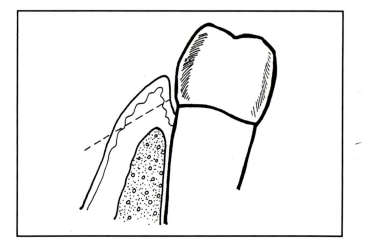

Fig. 1-1. A gingivectomy procedure to eliminate diseased or redundant tissue.

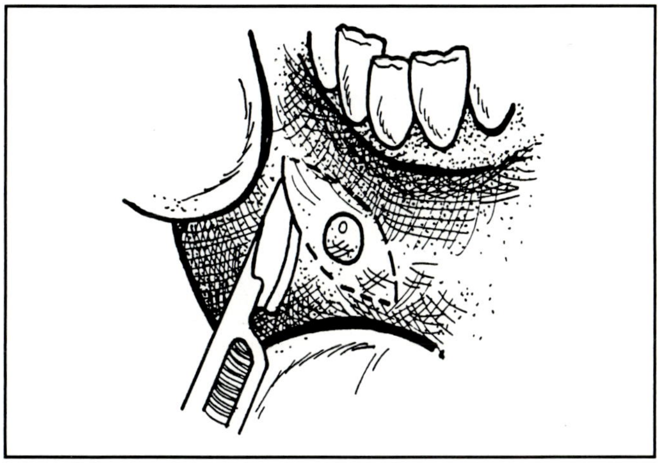

Fig. 1-2. Excision of a small, benign fibroma on the inner surface of the lip.

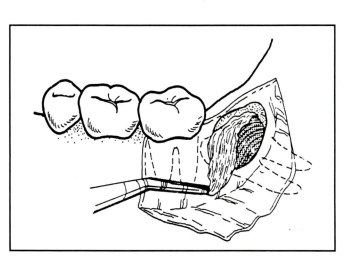

Fig. 1-3. Teasing out a follicle with a suction tip prior to its removal with a hemostat.

Mucoperiosteal Flaps

A flap (full-thickness or partial-thickness) is a portion of the attached gingiva and adjoining alveolar mucosa raised from underlying tissues by a surgical procedure. The base of the flap provides vascularity to the reflected tissue. The thickness of the flap will either be the total thickness of the tissue itself, from epithelial surface to bone (full-thickness), or the partial-thickness reflected to satisfy a specific purpose (a partial-thickness flap such as used with graft donor tissue).

A **full-thickness mucoperiosteal flap** is made as a means to an end, allowing the operator to accomplish definite surgical objectives. At the conclusion of a procedure, the flap can either be reapposed in the same position from which it was reflected or be repositioned apically or coronally. Full-thickness flaps permit the operator to perform such operations as 1) surgical crown lengthening, 2) apicoectomy, 3) alveoplasty, 4) osseous recontouring during periodontal surgery, or 5) "surgical" extraction of teeth with bone removal and/or sectioning. They provide access, protect soft tissue from trauma, and help control bleeding. *See Figs. 1-4 and 1-5.*

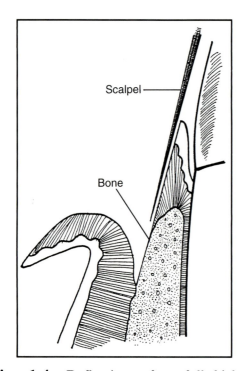

Fig. 1-4. Reflection of a full-thickness mucoperiosteal flap, exposing bone. Sulcular tissue is to be discarded.

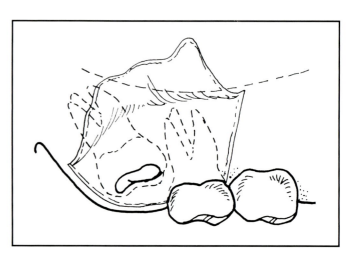

Fig. 1-5. Application of a full-thickness flap to provide access for the removal of a maxillary third molar.

This flap is generally developed from incisions made by the operator. The periosteal elevator lifts the soft tissue, including periosteum, from the bone by blunt dissection. The thicker the flap, the less pliable and flexible it will be. As thickness increases beyond two millimeters, the flap becomes increasingly difficult to manipulate.

Guidelines on the use of such flaps are few, but important:

1. Use sharp instruments and make clean incisions.
2. Include periosteum in the tissue to be reflected.
3. Allow a base wide enough to provide adequate vascularization.
4. Make flaps large enough to keep them from being stretched or torn.
5. Be familiar with the underlying anatomy in the area of the flap (such as the mental nerve).
6. Avoid tearing the flap or impinging on it during the procedure.
7. Place incisions where they will still be over bone during closure (they should be at least 4-5 mm from the edge of a defect).
8. When used for exodontia, releasing incisions should be placed one tooth away from the one being removed.
9. Close flap margins without pulling and without gaps.
10. After a flap is repositioned, apply gentle pressure on it for a minute or two to press out unwanted fluids and initiate a fibrinous adhesion.

The **partial-thickness flap** is made not as much for access as for accomplishing a specific purpose. It is made with sharp dissection instead of blunt dissection and divides gingival tissue at an intermediate level, thus leaving alveolar bone covered by soft tissue. *See Fig. 1-6.*

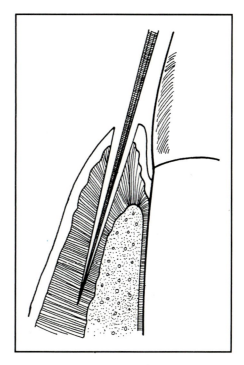

Fig. 1-6. Reflection of a partial-thickness flap. The position of the scalpel depends on what the operator wants to accomplish.

Bone Excision

Bone removal is an integral part of minor oral surgery. It is preceded by a full-thickness flap reflection which gives the operator good access to the surgical site and is a necessary prerequisite to performing such operations as exostoses excision, surgically lengthening crowns, recontouring bone damaged by periodontitis, accessing periapical pathology, and in many instances, removing teeth and roots. *See Figs. 1-7 to 1-12.*

The instruments used to excise bone are varied. In previous years, mallets and osteotomes were popular. Now handpieces and burs are more commonly used. Today's surgical handpieces in general practice may be either slow-speed (straight) or high-speed. In order to provide sufficient torque, straight handpieces should be capable of at least 20,000-30,000 rpm, not the mere 6,000-7,000 rpm used for restorative dentistry. Contra-angle attachments for straight handpieces can be used for surgery as the need dictates. High-speed handpieces should be of the type that do not force air into the wound, predisposing the patient to air emphysema. In the mandibular arch, this complication can lead to potentially life-threatening mediastinitis.

One underlying requirement with bone excision is that the bone not be overheated. For that reason, there must be adequate irrigation to dissipate the excess heat generated by friction. Irrigation fluids to choose from include tap water, distilled water, normal saline, and sterile saline. Saline, particularly sterile saline, is the recommended irrigation medium. If proper irrigation is not used and the bone becomes heated beyond a certain temperature, necrosis can result, with the possibility of subsequent infection, sequestration, and desquamation.

Methods of irrigation include:

- through a handpiece
- through a tube attached to the handpiece
- from an irrigation syringe
- from a three-way syringe

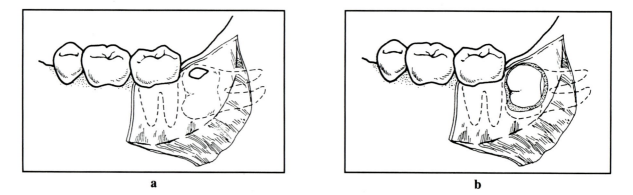

Fig. 1-7. a, A full-thickness flap is reflected, exposing bone over a mandibular horizontal impaction. b, With bone removed, the operator can section the tooth in preparation for withdrawal.

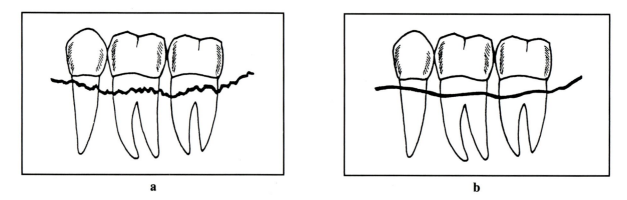

Fig. 1-8. a, Periodontitis can cause bone around the molars to become pitted and irregular. b, With osseous recontouring as depicted in this illustration, apical repositioning of the gingival tissue, and improved home care, the patient should be able to maintain a disease-free mouth.

Tooth Manipulation

Dental surgery frequently involves the manipulation of tooth structures in a precise manner. Some examples are listed below:

Section cuts are usually associated with exodontia, particularly impactions or the "surgical" removal of erupted teeth. Even when one is familiar with a certain type of section cut, if it is applied at the wrong angle or made to the wrong depth it may not accomplish the desired result. *See Figs. 1-9 to 1-11.*

Root amputation and hemisection are two examples of tooth manipulation requiring a knowledge of endodontics, periodontics, restorative dentistry, and exodontia. This includes familiarity with full-thickness flap procedures and quite often with bone recontouring.

Purchase points are utilized to effect the removal of teeth or roots. Several factors are essential for their success. First, they need to be placed adjacent to bone strong enough to be used as a fulcrum. Second, if the tooth has been sectioned, the purchase point should not be too close to the cut edge of the root (at least 2 mm away). Third, they should be approximately 2 mm deep. Fourth, forces should be applied in a direction that conforms with the anticipated line of withdrawal of the tooth. *See Fig. 1-12.*

Recontouring of crowns and roots is often necessary for them to conform to physiologic, anatomic, and/or surgical needs. Examples of procedures where recontouring is desirable are: free gingival grafts (root to be covered), root amputation, and hemisection.

Apicoectomy. Prior to a retropreparation and retroseal, the root apex is generally resected and beveled. *See Fig. 1-13.*

Replantation usually requires that an apicoectomy be performed.

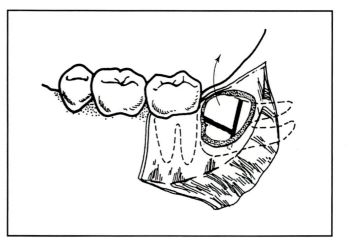

Fig. 1-9. Section cuts are utilized to allow the removal of this mandibular horizontal impaction. The more vertical cut is termed the "A" cut while the other one is referred to as the "B" cut.

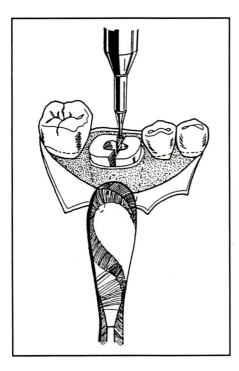

Fig. 1-10. A bur is being used to define the separation between the roots of this mandibular first molar prior to removing it in two parts.

Fig. 1-11. A straight elevator is inserted into the section cut of this mesioangular impaction. As the elevator is turned, the uncut tooth structure splits, thus completing separation all the way through the tooth.

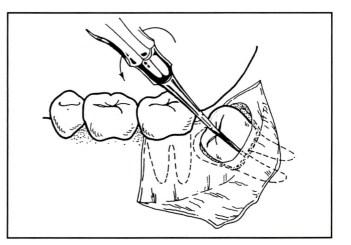

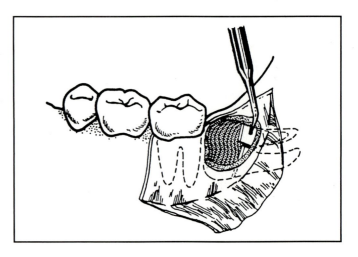

Fig. 1-12. With the crown of this horizontal impaction removed, a purchase point is placed in the superior root. An instrument uses distal bone as a fulcrum to dislodge the root.

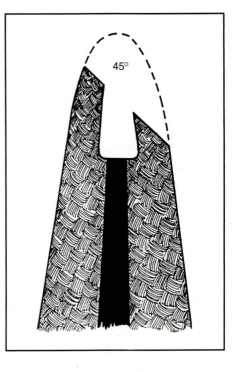

Fig. 1-13. In performing a retroseal procedure, approximately 2 mm of the root apex is resected. The tooth is beveled at a 45 degree angle and then a 2 mm deep retropreparation is cut into the apex in the long axis of the tooth.

CLINICAL CASES USING THE COMMON ELEMENTS

Free Gingival Graft

Figs. 1-14 through 1-17

COMMON ELEMENTS

- partial-thickness reflection
- soft tissue excision
- tooth manipulation

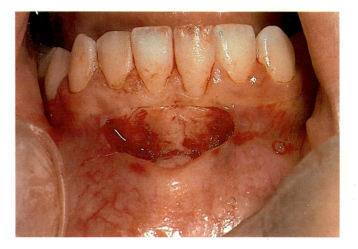

Fig. 1-14. Patient 1. An orthodontist requested that this patient have a graft labial to teeth #'s 24 and 25 prior to initiating treatment. This picture shows completed recipient site preparation which is, in essence, a partial-thickness flap reflection. Thin bleeding periosteum covers bone.

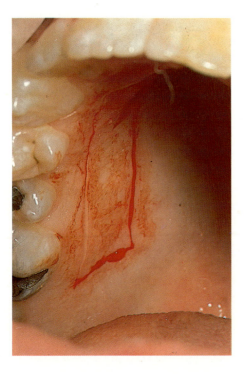

Fig. 1-15. Patient 2. A Bard-Parker #15 blade was used to define the outline of donor tissue for a free gingival graft. A partial-thickness reflection is about to be made about 1-2 mm under the epithelial surface. This is in stark contrast to the previously described partial-thickness reflection on the lower arch. The former was made next to the periosteum; this one was made several millimeters from the periosteum. The thickness of a graft depends on whether the operator is trying to cover a root surface (thicker) or simply creating additional attached gingiva (thinner).

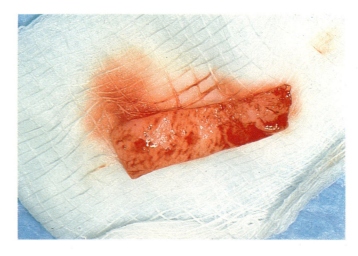

Fig. 1-16. Excised graft tissue.

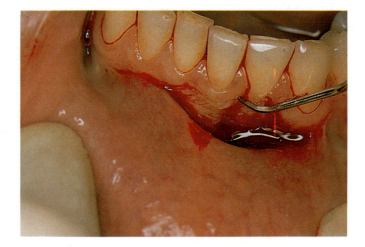

Fig. 1-17. Patient 3. In order to increase the predictability of root coverage with a free graft, the convex root surface is planed flatter (manipulated). This decreases surface area and eliminates surface contaminants that would compromise reattachment.

Surgical Crown Lengthening
Figs. 1-18 through 1-22

COMMON ELEMENTS

- full-thickness flap
- bone excision
- tooth manipulation (may be from trauma)
- soft tissue excision

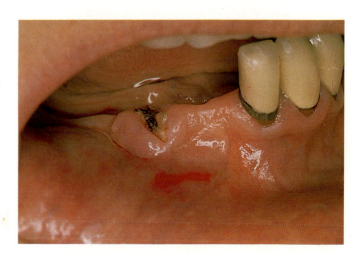

Fig. 1-18. Patient 1. The root shown in this picture is decayed to the bone level. The tooth is to become a partial denture abutment.

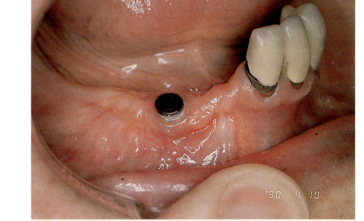

Fig. 1-19. Full-thickness flaps are apically repositioned after circumferential bone removal.

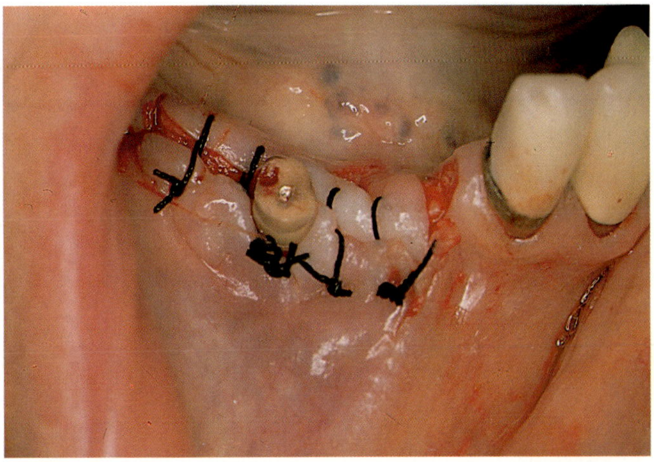

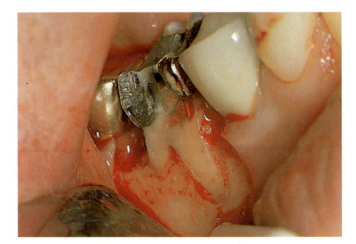

Fig. 1-20. A post and magnetic coping have been placed on the tooth. If this procedure were done on the palate, excess lingual tissue would be excised rather than repositioned.

Fig. 1-21. Patient 2. This tooth (#30) was recently treated endodontically and scheduled to be crowned, but the buccal side fractured before the work could be completed. Tooth #31 is not suitable as a bridge abutment. For that reason, the operator decided on surgical crown lengthening. Since the fracture extended apical to the bone level, a full-thickness flap was reflected and the bone smoothed down to the fracture line. In this case, the biological width of root surface required for normal periodontal healing was on the fractured portion of the root.

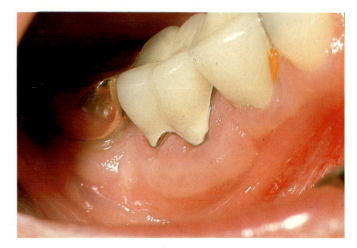

Fig. 1-22. After temporization for about two months, the tooth was crowned. The crown has a metal collar on the buccal that extends subgingivally into the sulcus. This is a seven year follow-up picture.

Apicoectomy and Retroseal
Figs. 1-23 through 1-25

COMMON ELEMENTS

- full-thickness flap
- bone excision
- soft tissue excision (lesion)
- tooth manipulation

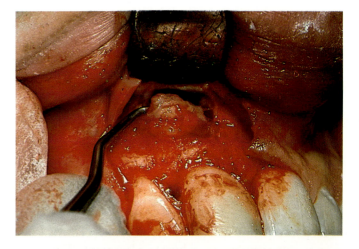

Fig. 1-23. Patient 1. Prior to performing an apicoectomy and retroseal operation, the operator curetted out fibrous granulomatous tissue from around the apex of this tooth. Pathology of this nature is not uncommon in long-standing infections.

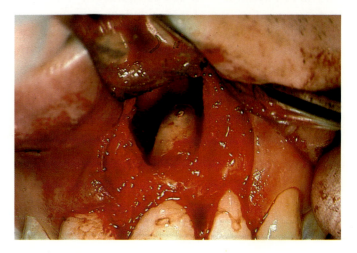

Fig. 1-24. As part of endodontic surgery, the root apex was resected and then beveled.

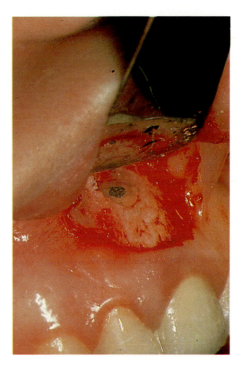

Fig. 1-25. Patient 2. Even though there were symptoms associated with this tooth that had been endodontically treated more than one year before, there was no apparent lesion or defect. The location of the apex was estimated and bone carefully removed to expose the end of the root. After the retropreparation was made, the apex was sealed with amalgam.

Intentional Replantation

Figs. 1-26 through 1-27

COMMON ELEMENTS

- full-thickness flap (cervical reflection)
- tooth manipulation

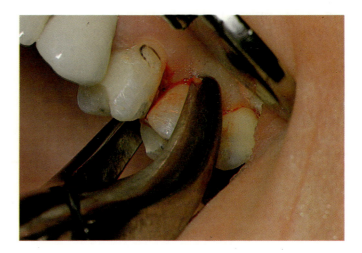

Fig. 1-26. A tooth is shown being extracted as part of an intentional replantation procedure. A cervical full-thickness flap was reflected prior to applying forcep beaks on the buccal and lingual.

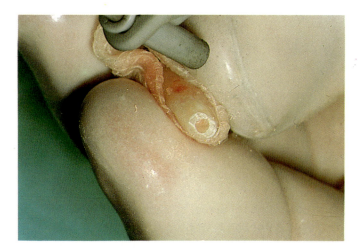

Fig. 1-27. Just as with a conventional apicoectomy and retroseal operation, with intentional replantation the root is resected. The amount cut away is still about 2 mm, but since visibility is not an issue, beveling is unnecessary. The retropreparation can be ideally made 3 mm deep.

Orthodontic Brackets on Unerupted Teeth

Figs. 1-28 through 1-30

COMMON ELEMENTS

- full-thickness flap
- bone excision (according to circumstances)
- soft tissue excision (follicle)
- tooth manipulation (bracket placement)

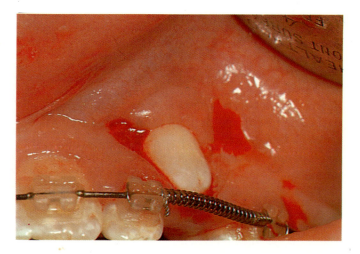

Fig. 1-28. Patient 1. This tooth in a 13-year-old patient is delayed in its eruption, requiring surgical assistance in order to complete the case in a timely fashion. Since the tooth was fairly close to the crest of the ridge, the operator merely made a semilunar incision and repositioned tissue apically to expose the crown's labial surface. No sutures were used, but gentle pressure was placed on the flap in its new position for a few minutes to initiate fibrin adhesion.

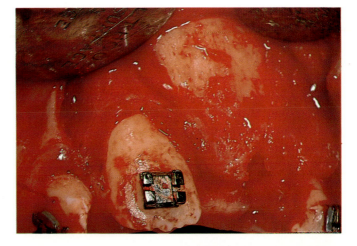

Fig. 1-29. Patient 2. A maxillary central incisor remains unerupted because of an existing supernumerary. To remove the extra tooth and access the central for bracket placement, a full-thickness flap was reflected, utilizing one releasing incision (triangular flap).

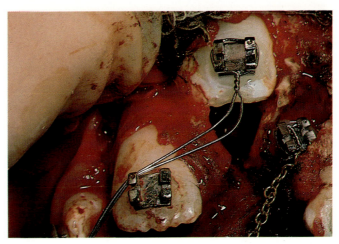

Fig. 1-30. This picture was taken after the mesiodens was removed and brackets placed on the lateral and central incisors. The flap will now be repositioned into its original location. Teeth will subsequently be pulled toward the archwire.

Alveolar Ridge Augmentation with Synthetic Bone
Figs. 1-31 through 1-33

COMMON ELEMENTS

- full-thickness flap (if needed)
- tooth manipulation (extraction)

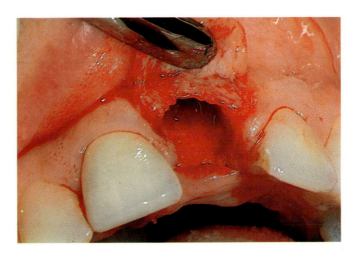

Fig. 1-31. Before extraction, pocket depths on this tooth measured 9 mm and a purulent exudate exuded from the sulcus when pressure was placed over the root. With the amount of bone destruction that had occurred, it was felt that normal healing would produce an excessively resorbed ridge not conducive to good esthetics. Four releasing incisions were made (two labially and two lingually) to facilitate more complete closure following the insertion of synthetic particulate bone.

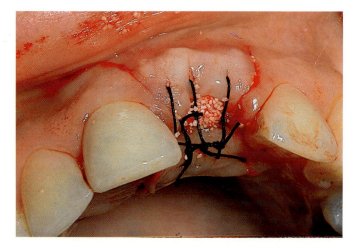

Fig. 1-32. With synthetic bone packed into the socket, buccal and lingual flaps were approximated as close to each other as possible.

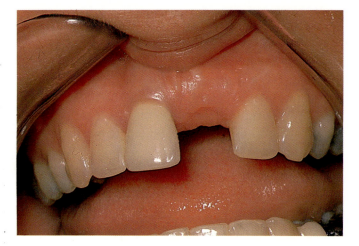

Fig. 1-33. Healing two weeks postoperatively.

Frenectomy Procedures
Figs. 1-34 through 1-36

COMMON ELEMENTS

- soft tissue excision (of frenum)
- partial-thickness flap (periosteum exposed)

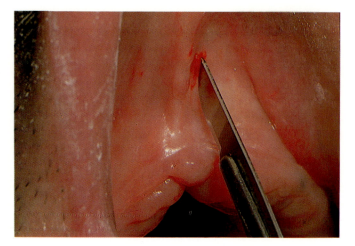

Fig. 1-34. To excise this frenum in an edentulous patient, incisions were made in the shape of a "V" — one on each side. While exerting traction on the frenum, it was released from the periosteum with a scalpel blade.

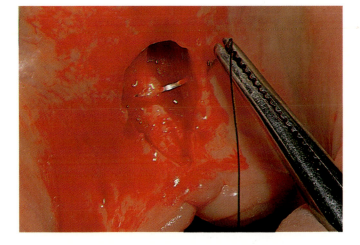

Fig. 1-35. Finally, the frenum was excised from the lip, creating the pear-shaped defect shown here. In this picture a suture is being placed at the level of the mucobuccal fold. Note that it passes through the exposed periosteum. This type of suture, binding soft tissue as high as possible to help prevent subsequent relapse, is termed an "anchor suture."

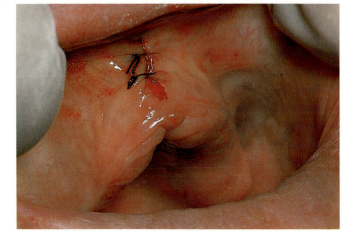

Fig. 1-36. Sutured case. Any underlying tissue that is not completely covered will be allowed to granulate in by secondary intention.

Small Lesion Excision

Figs. 1-37 through 1-38

COMMON ELEMENT

- soft tissue excision

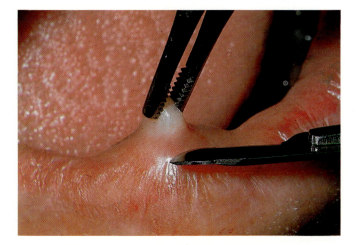

Fig. 1-37. Traction is placed on a small fibrotic lesion to allow a scalpel to more easily make elliptical incisions on either side of the growth.

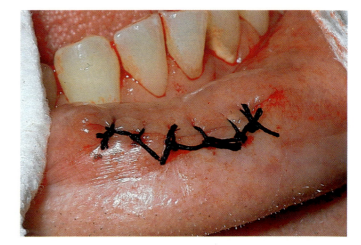

Fig. 1-38. Sutured case.

Fractured Root Removal

Fig. 1-39

COMMON ELEMENTS

- full-thickness flap
- bone excision
- tooth manipulation

Fig. 1-39. The tooth being extracted on this 60-year-old woman was nonvital and exhibited hypercementosis radiographically. Extraction was first attempted with conservative methods. As the tooth continued to fragment and resisted normal extraction efforts, a surgical approach was implemented. A full-thickness flap was reflected and buccal bone removed to within a centimeter of the apex.

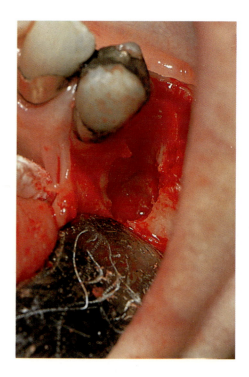

Impacted Third Molar Removal

Figs. 1-40 through 1-43

COMMON ELEMENTS

- full-thickness flap
- bone excision
- tooth manipulation (sectioning, purchase point)
- soft tissue excision (follicle)

Fig. 1-40. Patient 1. This mandibular third molar was partially erupted, which might lead some operators to think it could be extracted in a routine manner. In reality, this type often requires a flap broader in scope than the normal conservative cervical reflection, in addition to bone removal and sectioning. All of these steps were taken in this case. The tooth was then luxated. Next it was sectioned with a bur, after which a 301 elevator was used to complete separation. Part of the tooth is now being removed with a 151 forcep.

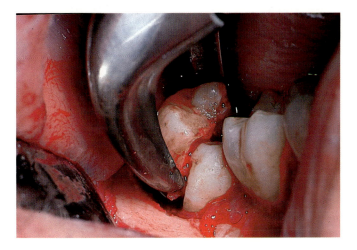

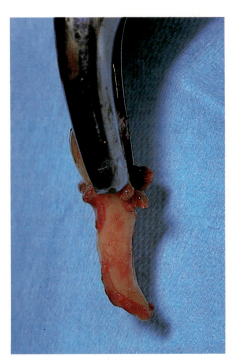

Fig. 1-41. Distal half of the tooth.

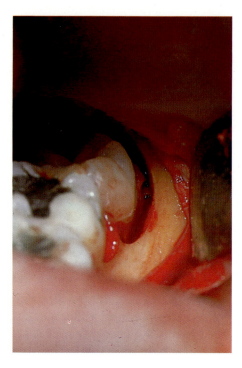

Fig. 1-42. Patient 2. This is a partial bony impaction. A flap has been reflected and a trough created buccally, extending distally.

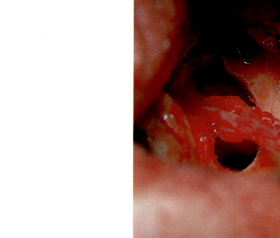

Fig. 1-43. *Continuation from Fig. 1-42.* The follicle is taken out after the removal of impacted teeth because of its predisposition to postoperative pathology.

Chapter 2

The Free Gingival Graft

INTRODUCTION

The free gingival graft is designed to establish a zone of attached, keratinized gingiva which is said to be "functionally adequate." While opinions vary on just how much attached gingiva is enough, it can be said that "a functionally adequate zone of gingiva is defined as one that is keratinized, firmly bound to tooth and underlying bone, and resistant to moving and to gaping when the lip is distended."[1]

DIAGNOSTIC CRITERIA

Table 2-1 lists items to consider when judging the adequacy of existing attached tissue and the need for more.

Table 2-1. Attached gingiva considerations

---

1. Width of existing attached gingiva

2. Presence of inflammation

3. Cause of the recession that may be present

4. Prognosis for additional recession

5. Age of the patient

6. Restorative or orthodontic treatment plan

7. Esthetic considerations

21

The etiology of gingival recession and subsequent mucogingival problems may include:

1. Tooth position. Teeth which are labially or lingually malpositioned or with prominent root surfaces may have decreased zones of attached gingiva or no attached gingiva.
2. Eruption pattern. A tooth may erupt with little or no attached gingiva or with a frenum pulling on the free gingival margin.
3. Periodontal pocketing which extends apically past the mucogingival line.
4. Gingival inflammation from plaque traps, poor home care, faulty restorations, or multiple causes.
5. Orthodontic tooth movement in areas of inadequate soft tissue.
6. Trauma from dental procedures, dental appliances, or chronic toothbrush irritation.

The free autogenous gingival graft is the most widely used, most versatile, and most predictable pure mucogingival surgical procedure in use today. The procedure was described as early as 1904, coming into generalized acceptance in the 1960s. Historically, the objectives for gingival grafting have varied. For this discussion, the primary objectives for free, autogenous gingival grafting are: (1) the prevention of additional gingival recession by increasing the width and improving the quality of attached gingiva, and (2) coverage of root surfaces which have been denuded through gingival recession.

Advantages and disadvantages of the procedure are given in Table 2-2.

Table 2-2. Advantages and disadvantages of the free gingival graft:

Advantages

1. It can be done for single or multiple teeth.
2. As a procedure to create or augment attached gingiva it is very versatile and predictable.
3. There is a relatively large source of donor tissue.
4. "Creeping attachment" may be expected during the year following surgery resulting in additional root coverage postoperatively.

Disadvantages

1. There are two surgical sites involved.
2. The palatal wound can be painful.
3. Color match can be difficult in areas of esthetic importance.
4. Root coverage is not always predictable.

Classification of Gingival Recession

Miller[2] has described four classes of marginal tissue recession:

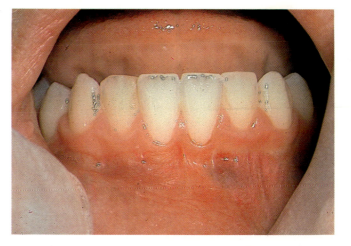

Fig. 2-1. Class I. Marginal tissue recession that does not extend to the mucogingival junction. There is no loss of interdental bone or soft tissue. Gingival augmentation is predictable. Root coverage is unnecessary.

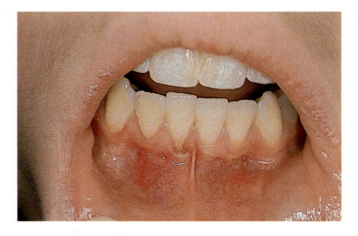

Fig. 2-2. Class II. Marginal tissue recession that extends to or beyond the mucogingival junction. There is no loss of interdental bone or soft tissue. Gingival augmentation is predictable. Some root coverage is likely.

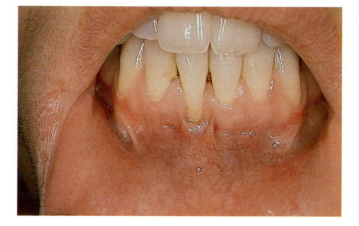

Fig. 2-3. Class III. Marginal tissue recession that extends to or beyond the mucogingival junction. Bone or soft tissue loss in the interdental area is present or there is malpositioning of the teeth. Gingival augmentation is predictable. Possible partial root coverage.

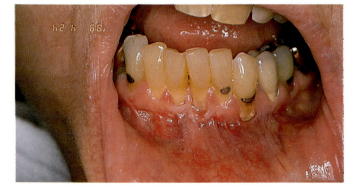

Fig. 2-4. Class IV. Marginal tissue recession that extends to or beyond the mucogingival junction. Bone or soft tissue loss in the interdental area and/or tooth malpositioning is severe. Gingival augmentation is predictable. No root coverage is expected.

Indications for the Free Gingival Graft

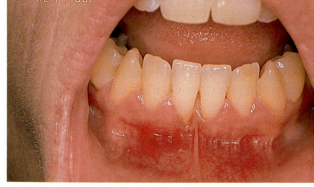

Figs. 2-5 and 2-6. One indication for the free gingival graft is to halt the progression of gingival recession.

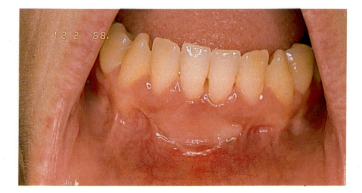

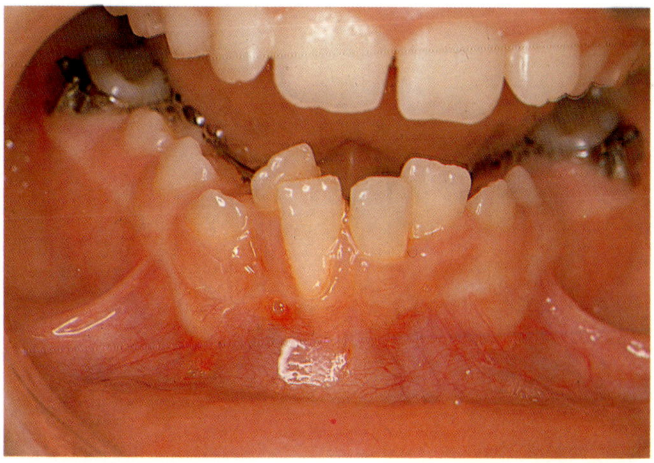

Fig. 2-7. A second indication would be to establish an adequate zone of attached gingiva prior to orthodontic treatment to prevent possible mucogingival problems or to supplement thin, delicate attached gingiva on prominent root surfaces,

Fig. 2-8. Same patient as in Fig. 2-7 above. Post-treatment picture showing healed graft in place,

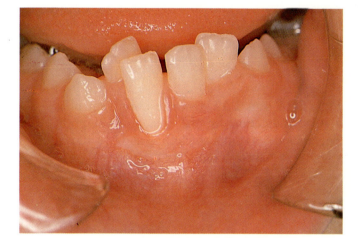

Fig. 2-9. Prior to restorative procedures which must be taken subgingivally,

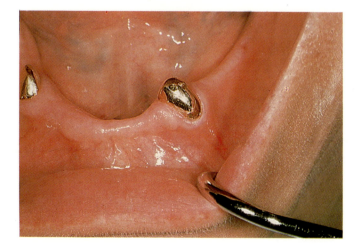

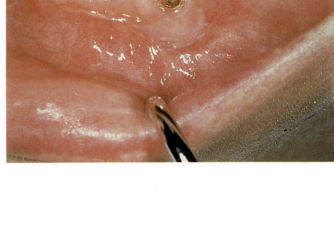

Fig. 2-10. Same patient as in Fig. 2-9. Post-treatment picture of healed graft.

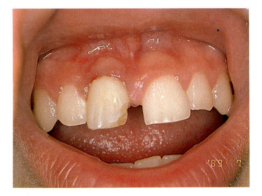

Figs. 2-11 and 2-12. Esthetic improvement is a third indication for the free gingival graft. This includes a) gingival clefting and b) gingival staining (amalgam tattoo, etc.).

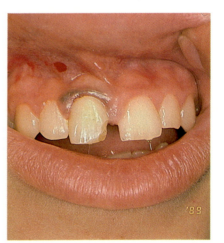

Figs. 2-13 and 2-14. A graft can be combined with a frenectomy procedure to prevent recurrence of frenum tension or to eliminate frenum tension on the gingival margin.

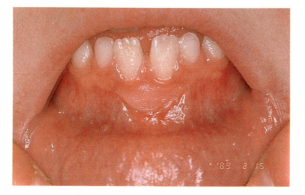

Knowledgeable, informed consent on the part of the patient is an important part of any dental procedure. The operator is obligated to provide information on the nature of the problem, treatment alternatives, and risk so that the patient can make an informed decision regarding treatment. A signed consent form is an integral part of this process. The following information may assist in designing a consent form along with the advice of an attorney or professional liability carrier.

Table 2-3. Example of Consent Form

Consent for Periodontal Surgery/Grafting

Patient: _____ **Date:** _____

Diagnosis: _____

Procedure: _____

1. I understand that the primary objectives of gingival surgery/grafting are:
   - to establish additional attached gum tissue to avoid further recession and loss of attachment.
   - to establish attached tissue more resistant to trauma, abrasion and home-care procedures.
   - to eliminate tension on the tissue margins which may aggravate tissue recession.
   - to eliminate periodontal pockets which may extend beyond the existing attachment gum tissue.

2. I understand that the secondary objective of gingival grafting is the covering of root surfaces already exposed by gum recession. I understand, however, that this is unpredictable and may not be possible.

3. I understand that, as with any surgical procedure, there are certain possible problems including:
   - adverse reactions to dental anesthetic
   - delayed healing
   - discomfort
   - infection
   - bleeding
   - altered tooth sensitivity to
   - altered sensations at the surgical sites   cold or heat

4. Alternative treatments, if any, have been explained to me.

5. The consequences of not treating this particular problem have been explained to me and may include:
   - further gum and/or bone recession, loss of support for tooth
   - periodontal pocket formation
   - inflammation or infection
   - tooth loss

6. I hereby consent and authorize Dr. _____ to perform periodontal surgery and all other necessary therapeutic procedures which have been described to me. I also consent and authorize the administration of such anesthetic or medication as may be deemed advisable for these procedures. If any unforeseen conditions arise during these procedures calling for the judgement of the therapist, I also authorize him to do whatever is advisable or necessary.

7. If the patient is under 18 years of age, his or her parent or guardian must sign below and agree to the foregoing on the patient's behalf.

_____
Signature of patient or guardian

SURGICAL TREATMENT

Table 2-4. Armamentarium

As with any oral surgical procedure, the best results are obtained when proper surgical principles are followed and proper instrumentation is used.

1. mouth mirror
2. periodontal probe
3. curette
4. surgical suction tip
5. 2x2 gauze sponges
6. local anesthetic: those with higher vasoconstrictor content preferred for hemostasis (epinephrine 1:50,000)
7. tissue pickups
8. scalpel with #15 blade
   - for recipient bed preparation, #15 blade is preferred
   - for donor tissue removal, either the #15 blade or Kirkland Gingivectomy knife works well.
   - Some operators prefer special instruments to remove the graft such as the Hu-Friedy Paquette Knife, the Gleason knife, the Deutch knife, or the XPO-111 knife, all of which allow the use of a razor blade loop, custom bent for the graft size, to make the incision.
9. needle holder
10. suture material: 5-0 with small needle is preferred
11. periodontal dressing material of choice
12. sterile foil: regular or adhesive
13. other items of personal choice

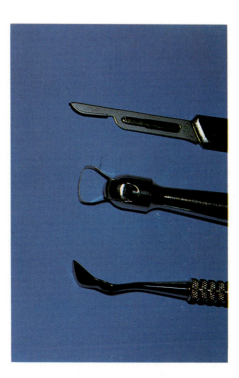

Fig. 2-15. Common instruments used for donor site surgery. **Top**, Bard-Parker scalpel handle with #15 blade. **Middle**, Paquette knife. **Bottom**, Kirkland gingivectomy knife.

Surgical Procedure

The surgical procedure for the free gingival graft may be divided into three steps: recipient bed preparation, donor site graft preparation, and graft tissue placement.

Recipient bed preparation

After suitable anesthesia, an incision is made horizontally, beginning laterally at the mucogingival junction to the level of the cementoenamel junction of the tooth being treated. The incision should extend one tooth laterally in each direction from the tooth being treated.

If there is some attached gingiva still present on the tooth, it can be left and the graft placed below this tissue to augment the existing attached gingiva. If no attached gingiva is present, the graft tissue will be the new marginal tissue.

With sharp dissection, a split-thickness flap is extended apically, preserving the periosteum. The mucosal flap generally retracts as the flap is created, but some mucosal tissue may be excised if additional space is required for graft tissue placement.

The connective tissue bed is prepared free of tissue tags or remnants of muscle fiber attachment. A smooth, thin connective tissue bed produces a better adapted, immobile graft result. If the periosteum is inadvertently perforated, it will probably not affect the success of the graft itself and will not require any changes in the procedure.

The denuded root surface is root planed to the cementoenamel junction to remove deposits and endotoxins which have penetrated the cementum. Root planing also reduces root prominence and produces contour corresponding to the surface of the connective tissue bed.

Donor site graft preparation

The palate provides a generous source of graft material, but tissue may be taken from any area with adequate attached gingiva, especially where it will not jeopardize adjacent teeth or other structures.

On the palate, the donor area should be posterior to the rugae but anterior to the second molar area (to avoid greater palatine vasculature). It can be close to the posterior teeth, but should not involve the free margin and sulcular tissue. The dimensions of the graft tissue can be determined by:

1. measurements with a periodontal probe
2. measurement with a periodontal probe, outlined on the palate with indelible pencil
3. constructing a template made of adhesive-backed foil or thin vaseline-coated cardboard, transferred to the palate

The apico-coronal width of the graft tissue should be about one third greater than what appears to be needed to compensate for anticipated shrinkage.

When donor tissue is taken with a scalpel, an incision is first made to outline the graft dimensions. This tissue is then undermined to a uniform depth of approximately one millimeter (or deeper for the purpose of root coverage[2]). When donor tissue is taken with a graft knife (Hu-Friedy Paquette) the blade is bent to the desired graft width and the length is determined by the insertion and removal of the blade in the tissue.

The incised tissue is placed on a gauze sponge wetted with saline. Adipose and glandular tissue, if present, should be removed from the connective tissue side of the graft to improve graft adaption and prevent any barrier to fluid infusion. The graft tissue is then trimmed to the dimensions of the prepared recipient site.

Donor site bleeding is controlled with manual pressure or a small amount of additional anesthetic with vasoconstrictor.

Graft placement

The graft tissue can be sutured in place using two or more interrupted sutures through the coronal aspect. If additional stabilization is desired, sling sutures either horizontally or vertically can be placed around the teeth and through the periosteum apical to the graft tissue. These sutures simply overlie the graft and maintain pressure against the recipient bed. It is unnecessary to suture the apical border of the graft or the mucosal tissue.

Once the graft is in place, pressure is applied for three to five minutes over the site using a moist gauze sponge. This provides:

1. an initial fibrinous adherence of the graft to the bed
2. prevention of blood pooling underneath the graft tissue
3. improved adaption of the graft tissue to the recipient bed
4. hemostasis

The graft site is generally covered with a protective dressing, although some operators choose not to do so. Such dressings may include a number of different substances such as those suggested in Table 2-5. Dressings and sutures are generally left in place from five to ten days.

Table 2-5. Graft Site Dressings

1. Periodontal pack
2. Metal foil with periodontal pack to prevent pack sticking to sutures
3. Stomahesive bandage
4. Orahesive bandage
5. Collagen or cellulose sponge
6. Biodegradable cyanoacrylate adhesive with or without amalgam squeeze cloth bandage

The palatal donor site, once bleeding is controlled, may be protected with materials such as those listed in Table 2-6.

Table 2-6. Donor Site Dressings

1. Periodontal pack
2. Stomahesive bandage
3. Orahesive bandage
4. Cyanoacrylate adhesive with or without amalgam squeeze cloth bandage
5. Clear acrylic palatal stent relieved over edges of the donor site to allow for anticipated swelling

Table 2-7. Free Gingival Graft Flowchart

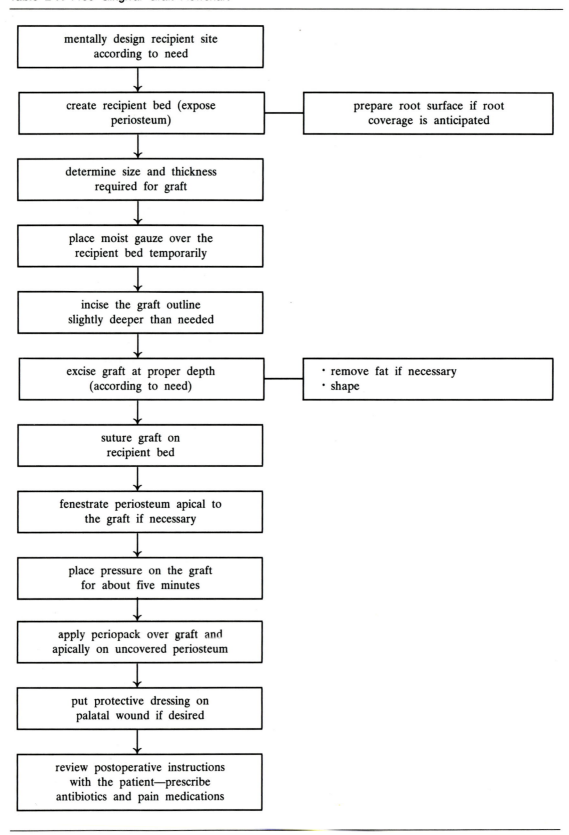

mentally design recipient site
according to need

↓

create recipient bed (expose
periosteum) ——— prepare root surface if root
coverage is anticipated

↓

determine size and thickness
required for graft

↓

place moist gauze over the
recipient bed temporarily

↓

incise the graft outline
slightly deeper than needed

↓

excise graft at proper depth
(according to need) ———
· remove fat if necessary
· shape

↓

suture graft on
recipient bed

↓

fenestrate periosteum apical to
the graft if necessary

↓

place pressure on the graft
for about five minutes

↓

apply periopack over graft and
apically on uncovered periosteum

↓

put protective dressing on
palatal wound if desired

↓

review postoperative instructions
with the patient—prescribe
antibiotics and pain medications

Table 2-8. Postoperative Instructions for Gingival Graft Patients

Written postoperative instructions should be discussed and given to the patient undergoing gingival graft therapy. The postoperative healing phase is in some ways unique.

1. The area from which the graft tissue was taken will feel uncomfortable for several days. The feeling is sometimes described as having been burned with hot food or hot drink.

2. Some bleeding for the first few hours following surgery is to be expected. If there seems to be more than just a small amount of oozing, pressure may be applied to the area of bleeding. If the bleeding is from the palate, apply pressure directly to the area with a damp wash cloth and finger pressure. If the bleeding comes from the area where the graft was placed, pressure may be applied to the outside of the face directly over the area.

3. Slight to moderate discomfort is normal following the surgical procedure. If medication has been prescribed, begin taking the medication before the numbness wears off, then continue to take the medication as needed every few hours for pain. To prevent nausea, do not take the medication on an empty stomach.

4. Try to stay with a soft diet for the first few days after surgery. Try to eat regularly during the day, but stay with foods that are relatively comfortable to chew.

5. Avoid rinsing your mouth the day of surgery. Rinsing generally will promote more bleeding the first day.

6. Lightly brush the areas which have been treated to keep those areas as clean as possible. Brush as well as you can comfortably.

7. The grafted area will undergo many changes during the first two weeks. Most noticeable will be color changes. It may first appear white and filmy, changing to red after a few days of healing. This is normal.

8. Your next appointment will be scheduled in five to ten days to remove the sutures placed during surgery. This will not be uncomfortable.

9. Follow-up visits after removing the sutures are important to follow the healing, insuring the very best result possible.

10. If any questions or problems arise, please feel free to call the doctor.

Free Gingival Graft Healing Phase

The graft must not be disturbed, especially during the first two days. During this time, plasma diffuses through a fibrin net in contact with the underside of the graft. Initial vascularization is present by about two days, but it takes seven days to provide a vascular network capable of adequately supporting the grafted tissue. Collagen attachment begins at approximately four days and becomes firm by ten days. The old epithelium becomes white and desquamates during the first three to five days. The new epithelium comes from surrounding tissue and may also proliferate from surviving basal epithelial cells.

New epithelium is evident by two weeks but ten to sixteen weeks are required for maturation. Keratinization takes approximately four weeks. Graft shrinkage is related to thickness—the greater the thickness the greater the contraction. Ridges and other irregular contours may be smoothed after several weeks with a gingivoplasty procedure if needed.

CLINICAL CASES
Case 1
Gingival Recession, Type I

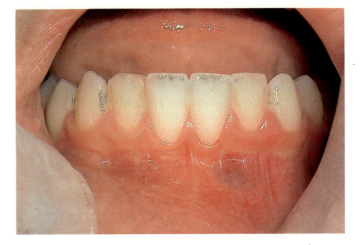

Fig. 2-16. Minimal zones of attached gingiva present labial to #24-25 with a high frenum attachment.

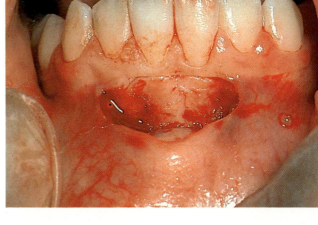

Fig. 2-17. Bed preparation preserves the small band of existing attached gingiva and eliminates the frenum. A gingival graft here will augment the zone of attached gingiva and prevent reattachment of the frenum.

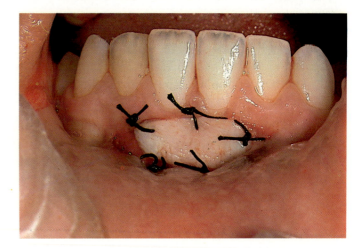

Fig. 2-18. The dimensions of the desired graft tissue are outlined on the palate using a piece of foil.

The graft tissue is undermined with the scalpel to a depth of approximately 1 mm, then gently retracted and lifted from the palate with tissue forceps. The tissue is transferred to a damp gauze sponge, trimmed of any adipose or glandular tissue and, if necessary, trimmed to the desired dimensions. It is sutured in place using interrupted sutures. Though used at the apical border of the graft in this case, sutures are not generally necessary apically.

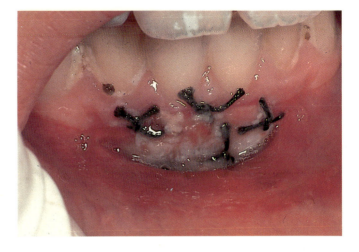

Fig. 2-19. Healing at one week—the time of suture removal. Surface epithelium desquamates, creating a white, yellowish or grayish film that rinses away with warm water. It is not necessary to repack this area. The patient may begin gentle plaque control procedures.

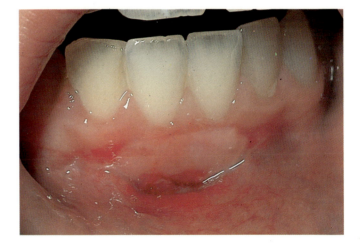

Fig. 2-20. Healing at four weeks postsurgery. While the graft is not yet mature and keratinized, the frenum has been successfully eliminated and a good zone of attached gingiva established.

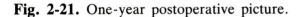

Fig. 2-21. One-year postoperative picture.

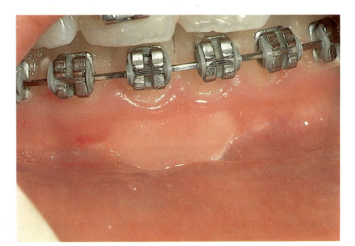

Case 2
Gingival Recession, Type II

Fig. 2-22. Teeth #24 and #25 both exhibit gingival recession. Tooth #24 has type I recession with some attached gingiva still present. Tooth #25 has type II recession with no attached gingiva present and three millimeters of root surface exposed. When tension is placed on the lower lip, the labial tissue distends from #25. The objectives of treatment are to:

1. Establish an adequate zone of attached gingiva.
2. Eliminate tension from the frenum.
3. Cover denuded root surface over #25.

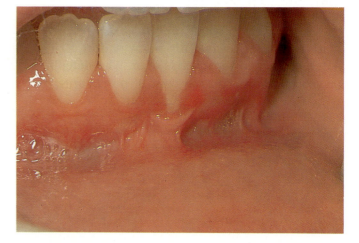

Fig. 2-23. Recipient bed preparation extends from the cementoenamel junction of the teeth coronally to the base of the vestibule on the apical edge. All tissue tags and muscle fibers are removed. The teeth are root planed.

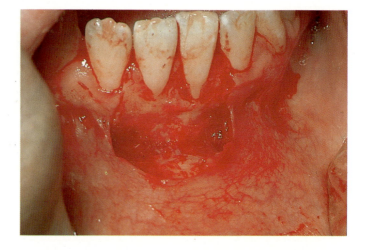

Fig. 2-24. Donor tissue is sutured laterally to secure it in place. A sling suture is placed through the periosteum apically, crosses the graft, and is sutured behind an incisor. This creates pressure to hold the graft tissue snug against the area where root coverage is desired.

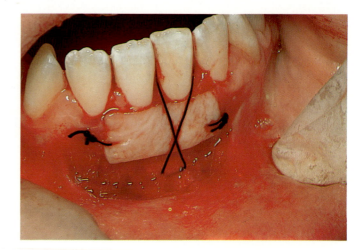

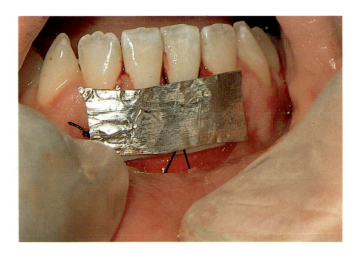

Fig. 2-25. Adhesive foil is placed over the recipient site to prevent the periodontal pack from adhering to the sutures.

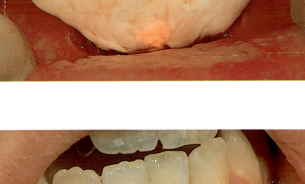

Fig. 2-26. A periodontal pack is placed over the recipient site, covering the foil and adapting interproximally. The palatal area is also covered with periodontal pack.

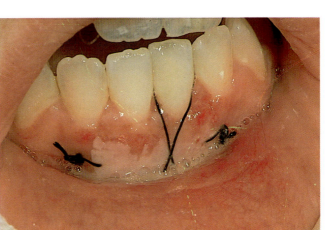

Fig. 2-27. Healing at one week. Sutures were removed at this time.

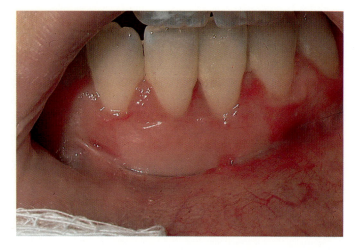

Fig. 2-28. Healing at one month, showing a good zone of new attached gingiva and coverage of the denuded root surface.

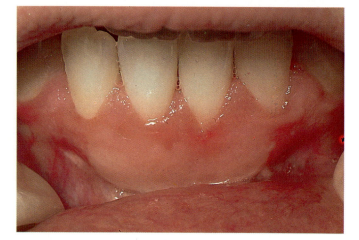

Fig. 2-29. Two-year postoperative picture.

Case 3
Gingival Recession, Type II

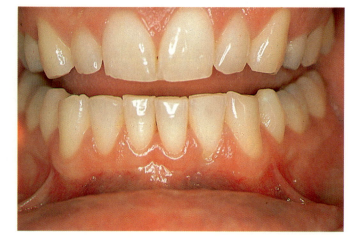

Fig. 2-30. Tooth #23 has no attached gingiva. Minimal zones of attached gingiva are present labial to #24 and #25. There is a high frenum attachment. Treatment objectives are to relieve the frenum, increase the width of attached gingiva labial to #23, #24, and #25, and to attempt root coverage on #23 to the cementoenamel junction.

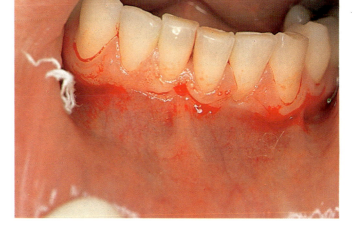

Fig. 2-31. The initial incision is along the mucogingival junction labial to #24 and #25, and to the cementoenamel junction of #23.

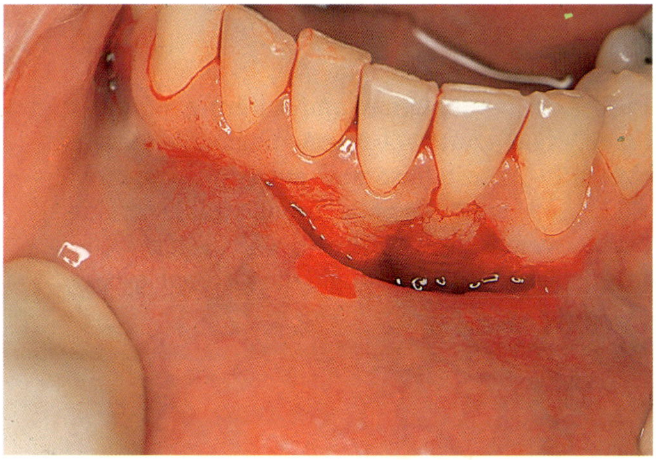

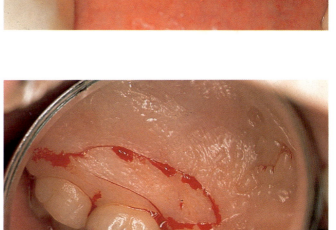

Fig. 2-32. Recipient bed preparation includes relieving the frenum. Tooth #23 is root planed from bone level to cementoenamel junction. The recipient bed is made as smooth as possible, removing any loose tissue tags and muscle fibers and leaving periosteum.

Fig. 2-33. Outline of donor tissue on palate made with #15 blade to depth of 1-2 mm. Dimensions are obtained by measuring with a periodontal probe.

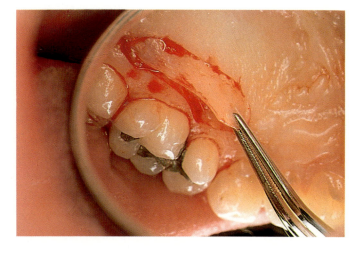

Fig. 2-34. Graft donor tissue is undermined with a #15 blade to a depth of about 1 mm generally, but 2 mm in the proximity of the root needing to be covered. Traction is accomplished with tissue forceps as undermining proceeds.

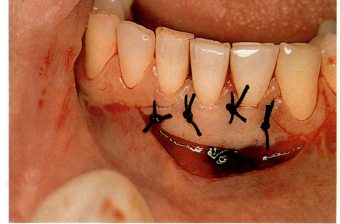

Fig. 2-35. Adaptation and suturing of graft tissue. The graft will augment gingival tissue over #24-25, establish new gingival tissue over #23, and create new marginal and sulcular tissue over the root of tooth #23. Interrupted sutures are placed through the coronal aspect of graft.

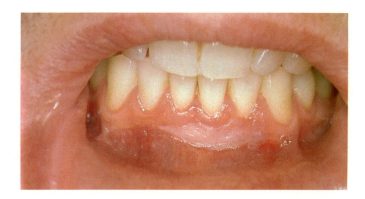

Fig. 2-36. Healing at one month post-treatment. The frenum was eliminated, a 6 mm zone of attached gingiva was established labial to #23-25, and the root of #23 was covered to the cementoenamel junction.

Case 4
Gingival Recession, Type III

Fig. 2-37. There is class III gingival recession labial to teeth #24-25. Recession extends apical to the mucogingival junction. There is malposition of tooth #25 and slight interproximal bone recession. Treatment objectives are to establish an adequate zone of attached gingiva for #24-25, to eliminate tension from the frenum, and to attempt root coverage.

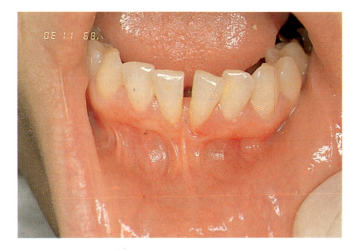

Fig. 2-38. Recipient bed preparation extending laterally for one tooth on either side, beginning at the mucogingival junction on adjacent teeth and extending to the level of the cementoenamel junction on #24-25. Teeth are root planed to the cementoenamel junction to eliminate deposits and endotoxins and to reduce root prominence.

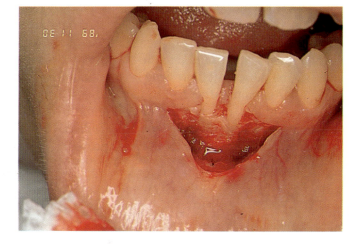

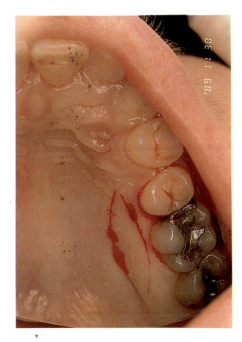

Fig. 2-39. The donor site is outlined with the dimension of the graft tissue needed using #15 blade. Dimensions can be determined with periodontal probe or with a foil stent.

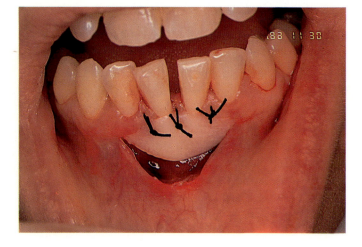

Fig. 2-40. Graft tissue adapted and sutured in place using interrupted sutures in the superior aspect of the graft. Graft tissue is brought to the cementoenamel junction of #24-25 to attempt root coverage.

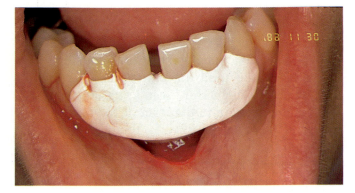

Fig. 2-41. A periodontal dressing is placed over the graft site. It is extended laterally beyond the borders of the graft, apically into the vestibule, and then adapted to·the interproximal spaces. The periodontal dressing is to remain in place approximately five to ten days, at which time the sutures can be removed. Premature loss of the periodontal pack generally will not adversely affect the success of the graft provided the area is not traumatized.

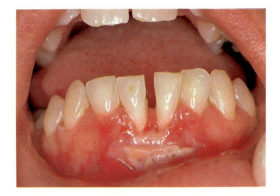

Fig. 2-42. Healing at one week (the sutures are removed at this time).

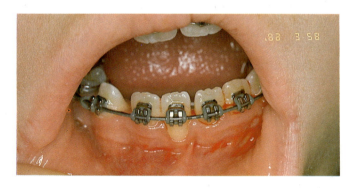

Fig. 2-43. Healing at six weeks posttreatment. A good zone of attached gingiva has been established over #24-25, tension from the frenum is eliminated, and partial root coverage has been obtained.

PROCEDURE OUTLINES

In this section, several different types of cases are shown along with their treatment objectives and a proposed graft outline designed to accomplish the desired objectives.

Case 1
Class I Gingival Recession on Erupting Dentition

Figs. 2-44 a and b. No attached gingiva on #25 with the free gingival margin at the cementoenamel junction. High frenum pull with tension on the papilla and marginal tissue.

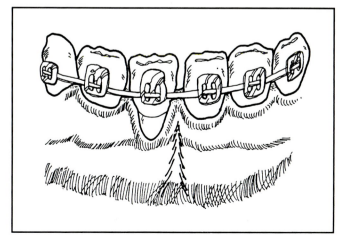

Fig. 2-44, c. Treatment objectives:

* Establish a good zone of attached gingiva over #25. You cannot even out the free margin because soft tissue will not adhere to enamel.
* Tissue levels will be uneven until further eruption of #24 takes place.
* The surgery will eliminate tension from the frenum.

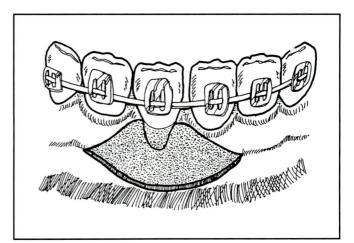

Case 2
Class II Gingival Recession

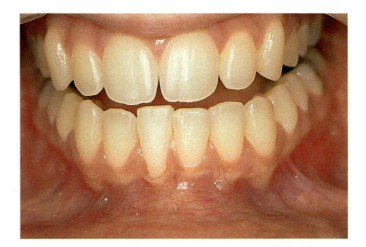

Figs. 2-45 a and b. No attached gingiva labial to #25 with tissue receded to the mucogingival junction.

Several millimeters of root surface exposed.

High frenum attachment with tension on papilla and marginal tissue.

No loss of interproximal bone or soft tissue.

Minimal attached gingiva on #24.

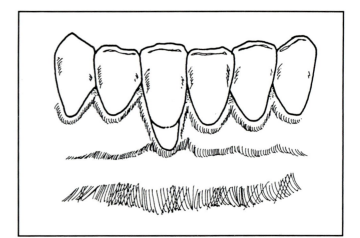

Fig. 2-45, c. Treatment objectives:

* Establish a good zone of attached gingiva on #25 and augment attached gingiva on #24.
* Root coverage on #25 back to cementoenamel junction may be possible.
* Eliminate tension from the frenum.

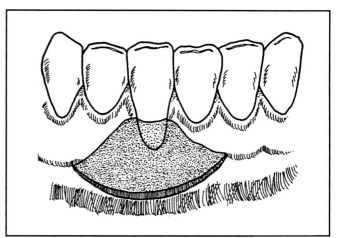

Case 3
Class II Gingival Recession

Figs. 2-46 a and b. No attached gingiva labial to #24 and #25 with tissue receded several millimeters apical to the cementoenamel junction.

Rolled mucosal tissue border.

High frenum attachment with tension on the papilla and marginal tissue.

No loss of interproximal bone or soft tissue.

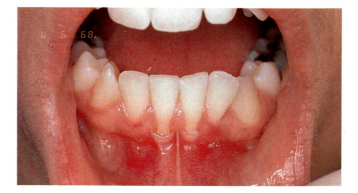

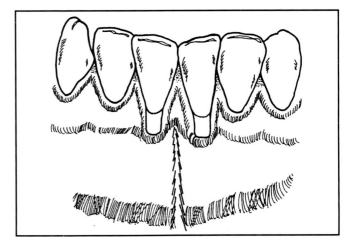

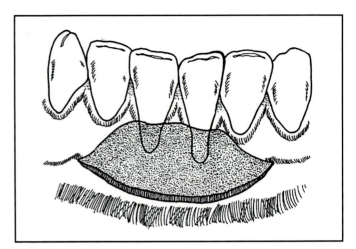

Fig. 2-46, c. Treatment objectives:

* Establish a good zone of attached gingival tissue over #24 and #25.
* Root coverage over #24 and #25 may be possible.
* Eliminate the frenum pull.

Case 4
Class III Gingival Recession

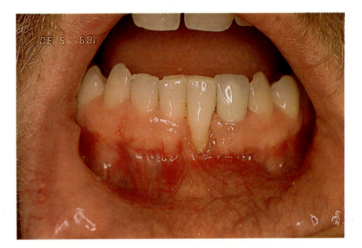

Figs. 2-47 a and b. No attached gingiva labial to #24.

Rolled mucosal tissue margin with several millimeters of root surface exposed.

Tooth #24 malposed. It is labially positioned with a prominent distolabial root surface.

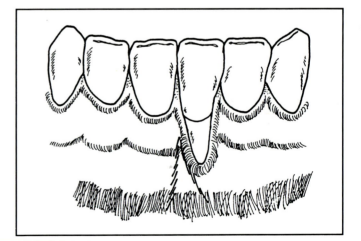

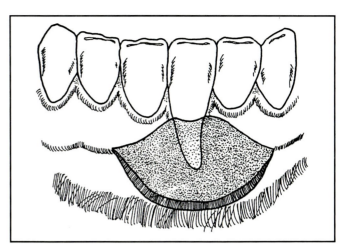

Fig. 2-47, c. Treatment objectives:

* Establish a good zone of attached gingiva.
* **Partial** root coverage may be possible. The width compromises the prognosis.
* Eliminate tension from the frenum.

Case 5
Class IV Gingival Recession

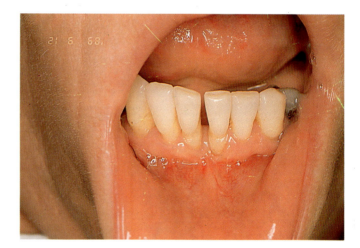

Figs. 2-48 a and b. No attached gingiva labial to #24 and #25, with tissue receded apical to the cementoenamel junction.

Several millimeters of root surface exposed.

High frenum attachment with tension on the papilla and marginal tissue.

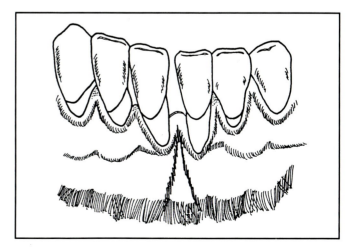

Fig. 2-48, c. Treatment objectives:

- Establish an adequate zone of attached gingiva for #24 and #25.
- Minimal root coverage is expected because of the extent of root exposure.
- Eliminate tension from the frenum.

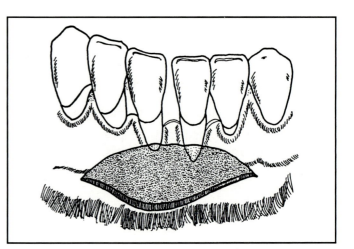

Case 6
Free Gingival Graft: Single Lower Incisor

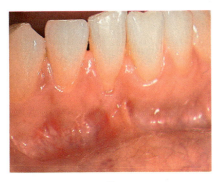

a

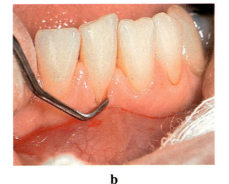

b

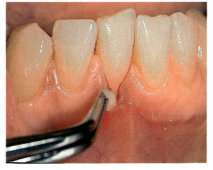

c

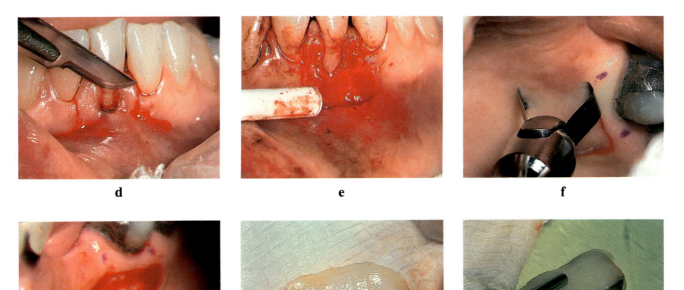

d

e

f

g

h

i

Fig. 2-49. a. Preoperative view showing deficient attached gingiva, muscle pull, and root exposure. Over the last few years, the case has been getting progressively worse. **b.** Root planing. **c.** Citric acid burnishing. **d.** Outline of incisions and beginning of epithelial peeling. **e.** Epithelium excised, exposing periosteum. **f.** Use of the Paquette knife to excise palatal tissue. **g.** Palatal wound. **h.** Donor tissue removed from the palate. **i.** The graft is refined in size and shape from the donor tissue. Tissue pickups and a new #15 blade are being used for this purpose. *(continued)*

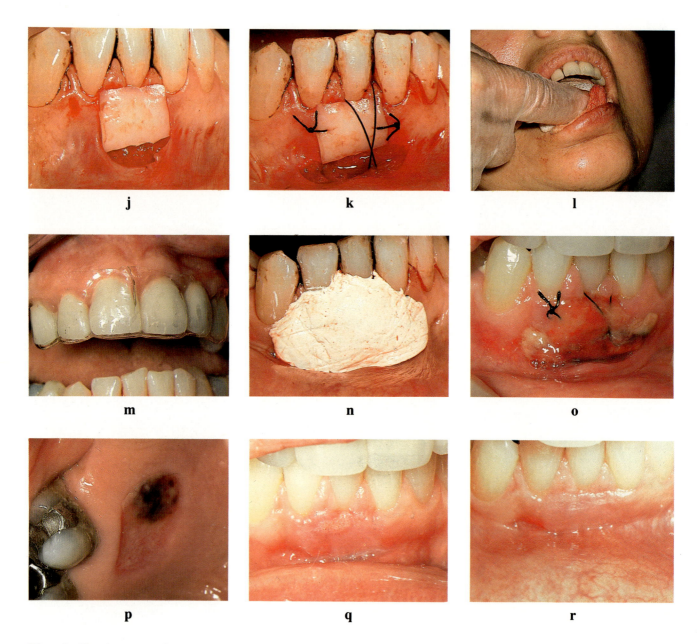

j

k

l

m

n

o

p

q

r

Fig. 2-49. *(continued).* **j.** Graft in position. It covers the root and proposed site of new attached gingiva. **k.** Graft sutured in place. **l.** Palatal bleeding is brought under control with local anesthetic (1:50,000 epinephrine) and gauze under pressure. **m.** A palatal stent made with a vacuum former is positioned in the mouth. It covers teeth to the facial gingival margin. The patient can eat soft foods with it in the mouth. Another design saddles the palate—not including anterior teeth. The wound can still be covered with topical anesthetic, cloth and cyanoacrylate, or other thin protective coverings. **n.** Graft covered with periopack. **o.** Five days postoperative. **p.** Palate at five days. **q.** Ten days postoperative. **r.** One month postoperative. A new zone of attached gingiva has been established, the muscle pull has been eliminated, and most of the exposed root has been covered.

References

1. Grant DA, Stern IB, and Listgarten MA. *Periodontics*. St Louis, Mo. The CV Mosby Co Inc. 1988.

2. Miller PD. Root coverage with the free gingival graft. *J Periodontol.* 1987;58(10):674.

Additional Reading Material

1. Harris J. Free gingival grafts by the general dentist. *Gen Dent.* 1981;29(2):146.

2. Dordick B, Coslet JG, and Seibert JS. Clinical evaluation of free autogenous gingival grafts placed on alveolar bone. *J Periodontol.* 1976;47:10.

3. Casullo DP, and Hangorsky U. The use of free gingival grafts in periodontics and restorative dentistry. *Compend Contin Educ Dent.* 1981;2(3):138.

4. Matter J. Free gingival grafts for the treatment of gingival recession. *J Clinical Perio.* 1982;9(2):103.

5. Epstein SR. The free gingival graft: goals of therapy and technique. *Compend Contin Educ Dent.* 1988;9(7):537.

6. Miller PD. Root coverage using a free soft tissue autograft following citric acid application. Part I: Technique. *International J Periodontics Restorative Dent.* 1982;2(1):65.

7. Brasher WJ, Rees TD, and Boyce WA. Complications of free grafts of masticatory mucosa. *J Periodontol.* 1975;46(3):133.

8. Miller PD. Root coverage using the free soft tissue autograft following citric acid application. Part II: Treatment of the carious root. *International J Periodontics Restorative Dent.* 1983;3(5):39.

9. Coslet JG, Rosenberg BDS, and Tisot R. The free autogenous gingival graft. *Dent Clin North Am.* 1980;24(4):651.

Chapter 3

Surgical Crown Lengthening

INTRODUCTION

The health of the periodontium is crucial in the prognosis for restored teeth, and many factors should be considered in determining the quality of soft and hard tissue surrounding such teeth. For example, some key factors are: the existence of inflammation or infection, the width of attached gingiva, muscle and frenum proximity, localized recession, hard tissue attrition and abrasion, sulcus depths (and whether or not there is bleeding on probing), the presence of bony defects, and the distance of anticipated restoration margins from the existing bone level.

Consideration of these factors is necessary to insure a long-lasting, quality restoration which is kind to supporting structures and can be maintained by the patient with reasonable home-care methods. Many teeth, however, present problems that lead to less than optimal conditions, making it impossible to adequately restore a tooth without some type of surgical intervention.

CASE SELECTION

At the gingival level, the tooth-periodontium interface is a functional unit consisting of three parts:

1. A free gingiva/anatomical sulcus that is 1 + mm in depth.

2. Epithelial attachment/junctional epithelium approximately 1 mm wide.

3. Connective tissue attachment—generally considered to be greater than 1 mm but less than 2 mm in width.

The combined dimensions of the epithelial attachment and the connective tissue attachment are termed the "biologic width" of the tooth (*see Fig. 3-1*). This width is generally considered to be approximately 2.04 mm along the root surface of a healthy tooth, but may be as much as 2.87 mm.

Dental restorations of any kind must not violate or impinge upon this "biologic width." When a restoration margin is placed closer than 2 mm to the crestal bone, this width is violated and periodontal problems will result, including chronic inflammation, soft tissue hyperplasia, and subsequent localized periodontitis. There may also be tooth hypersensitivity and pain from adjacent tissues.

Biologic Width

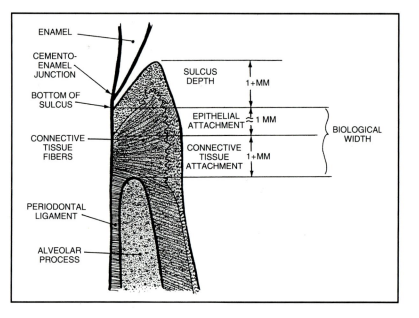

Fig. 3-1. An illustration of the biologic width.

From a periodontal standpoint, the most desirable restorative margins are supragingival. Unfortunately, this is not always possible and margins are extended into the gingival crevice for such reasons as improved esthetics, subgingival caries, and a need for greater retention.

In preparing a tooth for an intracrevicular margin, there should be a pre-existing healthy sulcus depth of at least 1.5 mm to 2.0 mm in order to allow the restoration margin to be covered by free gingiva while at the same time not impinging on the "biologic width." If sulcus depth is less than 1.5 mm, it is not reasonable to expect a healthy intracrevicular margin.[1] There should be at least 1 mm of tooth structure coronal to the base of the sulcus to prevent impingement of the restoration on the soft tissue attachment.[2]

When the requirements for adequate tooth structure and adequate periodontal attachment cannot both be met, the tooth needs clinical crown lengthening. For this discussion, only the surgical choices will be mentioned.

Indications for Treatment

Table 3-1. Indications for Surgical Crown Lengthening

1. To reduce hyperplastic gingiva, thereby improving esthetics and access for plaque control (Fig. 3-2).
   - gingival hyperplasia: inflammatory, familial, or medication-induced
   - altered or delayed passive eruption, gingival deformity

2. For tooth overeruption:
   - to establish gingival margins and contours harmonious with those of adjacent teeth while correcting the occlusal plane (Fig. 3-3).

3. For crown fractures in proximity to the gingival margin or at or below the osseous crest (Fig. 3-4).

4. For interproximal caries, cervical caries, or external root resorptive lesions near the osseous crest (Figs. 3-5 to 3-7).

5. For pin/core or post/core buildups of broken-down teeth with margins near the osseous crest (Figs. 3-8 to 3-9).

6. For the repair of post or pin perforations within the periodontal attachment or osseous structures.

7. To increase the length of short clinical crowns, thus providing better retention for restorations and clasps.

8. To revise tooth preparations carrying margins further apically past subgingival ledges.

9. To increase the length of the clinical crown when the loss of tooth structure has occurred from occlusal wear or chemical, abrasive, and traumatic factors (Fig. 3-10).

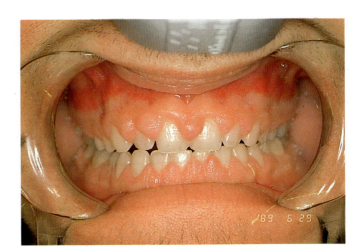

Fig. 3-2. Hyperplastic gingiva.

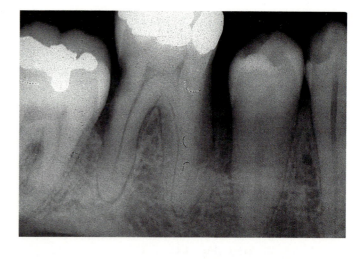

Fig. 3-3. Tooth overeruption.

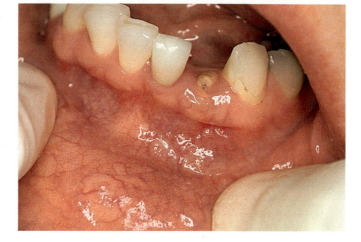

Fig. 3-4. Crown fracture in proximity to the gingival margin.

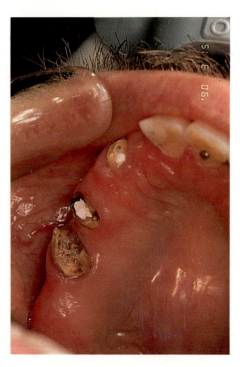

Fig. 3-5. Caries extending subgingivally to the osseous crest in prospective abutment teeth.

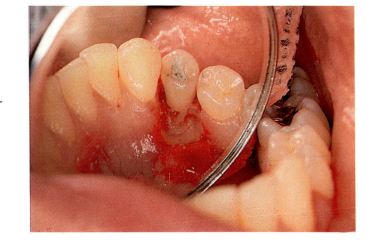

Fig. 3-6. External resorptive lesion—mesiolingual line angle at osseous crest.

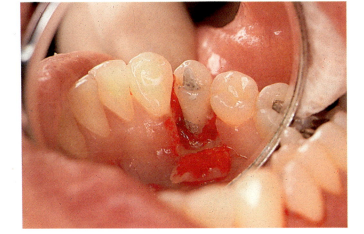

Fig. 3-7. Repair of resorptive lesion.

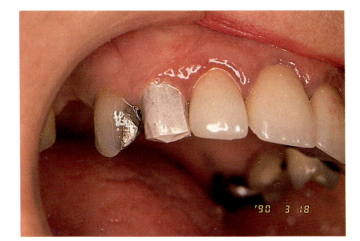

Figs. 3-8 and 3-9. Post/core buildup of lateral incisor which extends subgingivally on all surfaces.

Fig. 3-9.

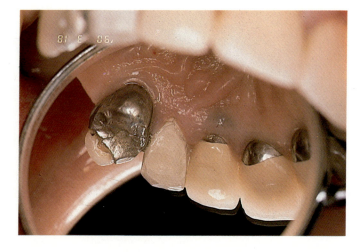

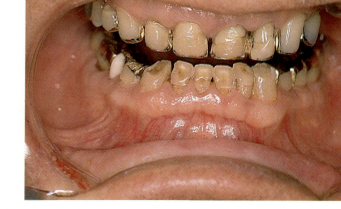

Fig. 3-10. Loss of tooth structure requiring increase of the length of the clinical crown.

Because crown lengthening involves a surgical procedure and requires an increased level of awareness and commitment on the part of both the dentist and patient, there are many factors which must be considered before making the decision to treat a tooth (see Table 3-2).

Before treatment begins, certain elements should be considered for each tooth involved. Both the dentist and the patient should feel that this therapy is the best treatment choice available. Treatment results must be functionally, biologically, and cosmetically acceptable.

There are three criteria which must be met for a crown lengthening procedure to be considered successful.[3] These include:

1. The exposure of adequate sound supragingival tooth structure for the placement of the restorative margins.

2. The presence of at least a 3-mm supraalveolar zone necessary to allow establishment of the "biologic width" and sulcus. (3 mm from crestal bone to restorative margin).

3. The presence of sufficient bone to provide adequate support for the restored tooth.

Table 3-2. Considerations for Surgical Crown Lengthening

1. Strategic position of the tooth in the arch.

2. Anticipated posttreatment esthetics.

3. The condition of adjacent teeth. Crown lengthening surgery will also affect adjacent teeth through physiologic remodeling.

4. Anticipated final crown/root ratio and anticipated tooth stability.

5. Amount of remaining attached gingiva.

6. Root dimensions. Long, tapering roots provide better support and prognosis for success than short, conical roots.

7. Location of furcations. Surgical therapy should not jeopardize furcations.

8. Root trunk. A long root trunk from the cementoenamel junction to the furcation provides a better prognosis than a short root trunk with less possibility of involving the furcations.

9. Adjacent root proximity. Surgical therapy should not adversely affect periodontal support of adjacent teeth.

10. Anatomic limitations of surgery.

11. The patient's commitment to this level of care.

Treatment Sequence

As in all aspects of dental care, crown lengthening procedures should follow an established, well defined sequence of treatment.

Table 3-3. Treatment Sequence for Surgical Crown Lengthening

1. Clinical and radiographic examination

2. Treatment plan presentation, informed consent

3. Provisional restoration as needed to control caries, facilitate plaque control, and prevent tooth migration

4. Inflammation avoidance through plaque control, scaling, and root planing

5. Surgical procedure

6. Healing phase

7. Final evaluation of surgery

8. Restorative therapy

Armamentarium for Surgical Crown Lengthening

Though there are many individual preferences for instruments, the general armamentarium for this procedure will include:

dental mirror	periosteal elevator	periodontal diamond stones
periodontal probe	tissue retractor	carbide burs
explorer	scalers	perio bone chisels (several kinds)
scalpel handle and blades	curettes	hemostat
gingivectomy knife	soft tissue nipper	needle holder
	scissors	suture
	periodontal dressing	

SURGICAL OPTIONS

Crown lengthening may involve the following types of procedures:

1. Gingivectomy by external bevel incision:

    a) when defects to be restored are suprabony

    b) when there is a wide, even redundant zone of attached gingiva present

    c) when the sulcus is deepened by soft tissue pocketing—no osseous defects are present.

2. Periodontal flap procedures:

    a) periodontal flap, apically repositioned

    • when lesion to be restored is 3 mm or more coronal to bony crest

    • when osseous recontouring is not needed

    b) periodontal flap, ostectomy, flap apically repositioned

    • when lesion to be restored is less than 3 mm from the bony crest or is below the bony crest

    • when physiologic osseous recontouring is required

    c) palatal area may involve an internal inverse bevel rather than apical repositioning

Crown lengthening is most often done using a periodontal flap because of better preservation of attached gingiva, better access and visibility of the tooth surfaces and osseous contours, and better flexibility in relocating the position of the gingival margin.

Crown Lengthening: Gingivectomy by External Bevel Incision

Gingivectomy is usually the procedure of choice when there is gingival hyperplasia: the sulcus is deepened by soft tissue pocketing; a wide, even redundant zone of attached gingiva exists; no osseous defects are present; and the defects to be restored are suprabony.

Figure 3-11 presents a case with moderate gingival hyperplasia in the anterior areas following orthodontic treatment. Inflammation has been controlled with only minimal soft tissue shrinkage. Gingival contours are unhygienic and unesthetic. Physiologic contours can be reestablished through gingivectomy.

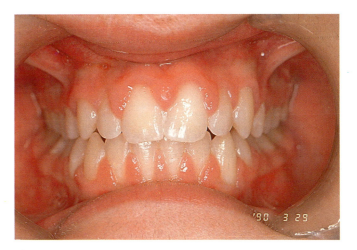

Figs. 3-11 and 3-12. Moderate gingival hyperplasia.

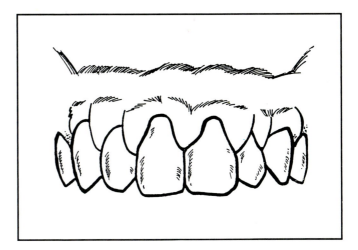

After suitable anesthesia is achieved, the initial incision is made buccally and lingually using a steep, external bevel. It extends from the bottom of the sulcus, progressing apically through the keratinized tissue and is then carried laterally from the surgical site to permit a smooth, blended soft tissue contour (Figs. 3-13, 3-14). Consider a scalpel, Kirkland knife, or other similar instrument for initial incisions. Electrosurgery is also frequently used.

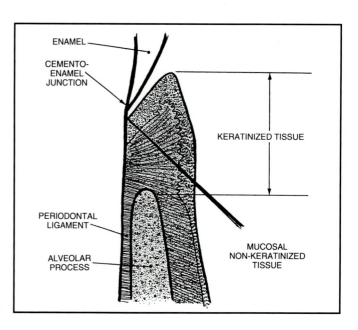

Fig. 3-13. Gingivectomy incision, external bevel.

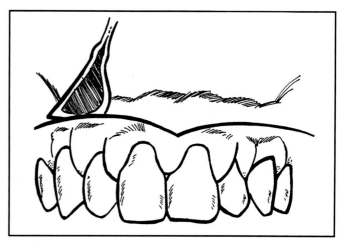

Fig. 3-14. Facial view of gingivectomy incision.

The incisions are then carried between the teeth using an interproximal knife (Blake, Goldman Fox, Orban, etc.), connecting the buccal and lingual incisions. Once these incisions are completed, the relieved tissue is removed with a scaler or curette.

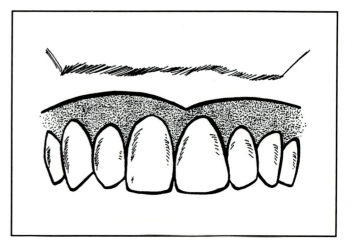

Fig. 3-15. View following the removal of excised tissue, debridement, contouring, and root planing.

The tooth or root surfaces are planed to remove deposits, contaminated cementum, and to achieve as smooth a surface as possible. The soft tissue surface is debrided, smoothed, and blended with adjacent tissue using the surface of a scalpel, soft tissue nippers, or rotary diamond stones.

The case is evaluated to be certain that tissue contours are acceptable, the wound surface is free of epithelial tags, tooth surfaces are clean, and that the lesion which is to be restored is accessible.

A periodontal dressing is usually applied. Dressings are removed 5 to 10 days postoperatively, at which time the teeth are polished. Plaque control measures are begun, which may include rinsing with chorhexidine until epithelialization is complete.

By three weeks, the wound surface is again covered with epithelium, and by 2 to 3 months, keratinization of the epithelium and maturation of the connective tissue is complete. The case is then ready for restorative treatment.

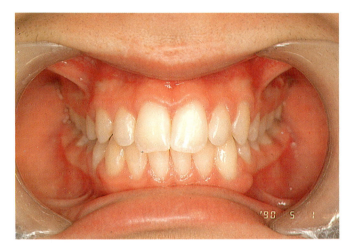

Fig. 3-16. Completed healing with physiologic contours restored.

Crown Lengthening by Periodontal Flap, Osseous Resection, and Flap Repositioning

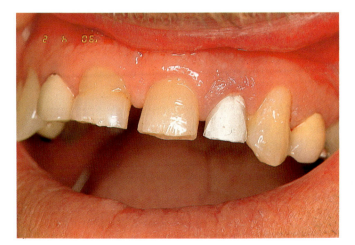

Figs. 3-17 and 3-18. Treating a maxillary lateral incisor which has decayed through tooth structure at the gingival level under an existing crown. After endodontic therapy and caries removal, no clinical crown remained above the gingiva. A post and core buildup has been done, but the core material is subgingival. No dentin surface is present on which to finish the crown margin.

Fig. 3-18.

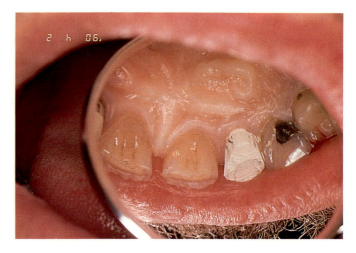

Fig. 3-19. Following adequate anesthesia, an internal bevel incision is made in the marginal gingiva and a full-thickness mucoperiosteal flap is raised buccally and lingually. The flap should also provide access to the interproximal surfaces. The internal bevel incision thins the marginal tissue for better postoperative adaptation and preserves keratinized epithelium. Vertical releasing incisions may be used as needed to provide adequate access.

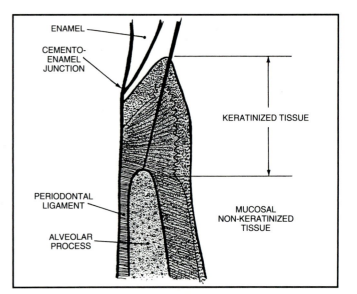

Fig. 3-20. After flap reflection, we see very little root surface between the buildup margin and the osseous crest. Adequate root surface must be present to allow for adequate "biologic width" and sulcus depth in which to place the restoration margin.

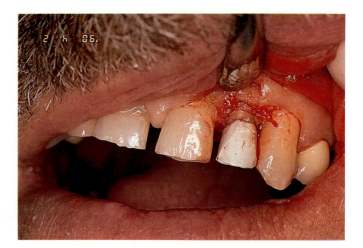

Fig. 3-21. Bone is removed at the alveolar crest to give the necessary three millimeters. This provides:

1-2 mm for connective tissue fibers

1 mm for junctional epithelium

1 mm for the reformation of the gingival sulcus (as the sulcus matures, this depth will increase)

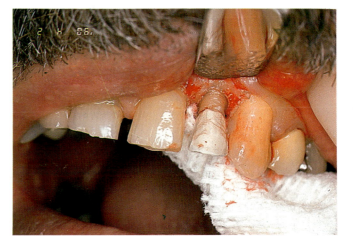

Fig. 3-22. Bone can be removed with rotary instruments and copious irrigation, or with hand instruments. Bone should be removed in all dimensions—buccal, lingual, and interproximal, establishing a physiologic contour.

When osseous recontouring is completed and gingival tissue repositioned, there should be at least 1 mm of sound tooth structure supragingivally. The flap is sutured into position at the tooth/bone junction. The clinical sulcus will reform through coronal migration as the tissue matures.

A periodontal dressing is applied to help stabilize the flap placement and for patient comfort. Sutures can be removed in 5 to 10 days. Plaque control measures should be initiated.

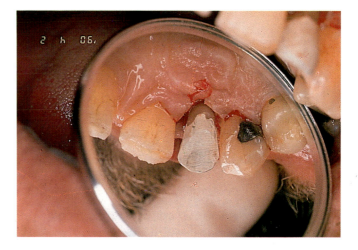

SUMMARY OF IMPORTANT CONSIDERATIONS

Additional suggestions for the surgical procedure

- bony margins should be thin
- grooves or spillways may be created as needed
- blend the ostectomy over adjacent teeth to form a flowing contour
- do not leave widow's peaks in interproximal areas—trim with chisel
- treat periodontal problems concurrently, if present
- all surfaces should be root planed and smoothed

Healing phase considerations

- suture removal at 5 to 10 days
- plaque control measures should begin immediately
- the tooth should have an adequate buildup or provisional restoration
- soft tissue maturation and repair is complete by 4 to 5 weeks postoperatively
- firm epithelial and connective tissue attachments are present 8 to 12 weeks postoperatively
- The tooth may be restored in the conventional manner after three months

Does the healed surgical case meet the criteria for success in crown lengthening?

- adequate tooth structure is present for the placement of restorative margins
- at least 3 mm of supraalveolar tooth structure needed to reestablish "biologic width" is present
- there is sufficient bone remaining to provide adequate support for the restored tooth.

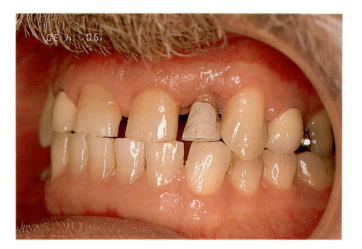

Figs. 3-23 and 3-24. The presence of these elements will provide a functionally, biologically, and cosmetically acceptable result.

Fig. 3-24.

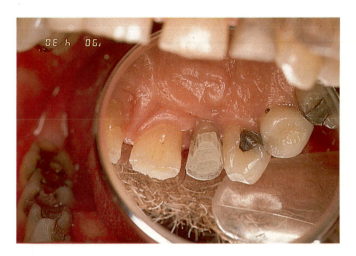

Table 3-4. Surgical Crown Lengthening Flowchart

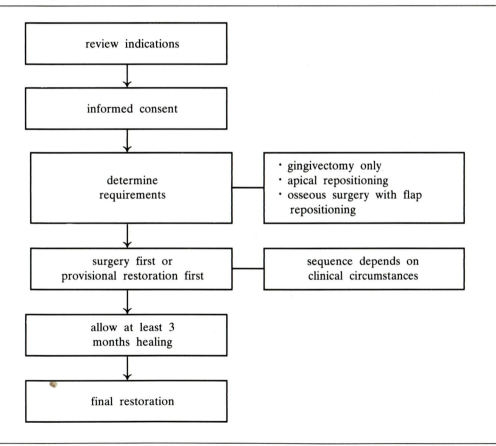

CLINICAL CASES
Case 1
Treatment of Dilantin Hyperplasia with Electrosurgery Gingivectomy

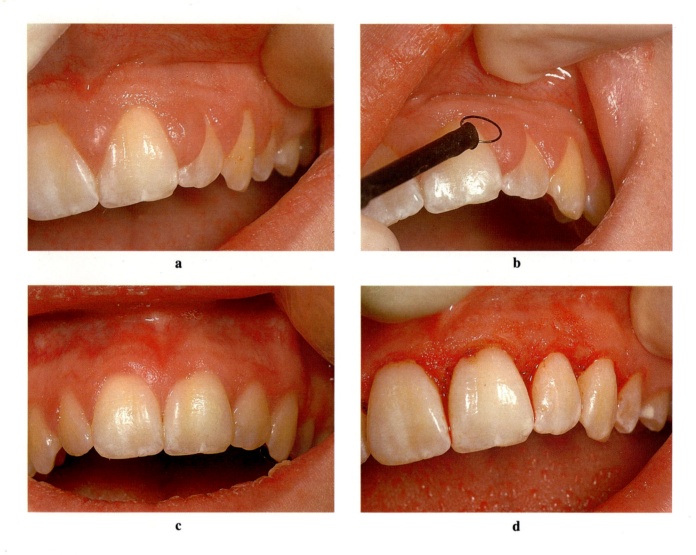

Fig. 3-25. a. This fifteen-year-old girl is taking Dilantin for epileptic seizures. Periodically, soft tissue around the teeth hypertrophies to the extent that it needs to be removed. **b.** In this instance, an electrosurgery loop is going to be used to excise redundant tissue. **c.** The bulk of the tissue has been removed. Some refinement can be performed with a periodontal curette. **d.** Early postoperative healing.

Case 2
Maxillary Lateral Incisor Obliquely Fractured

Crown lengthening was accomplished with a flap approach, osseous recontouring, and lingual gingivectomy of the flap. A provisional restoration was made at the time of surgery.

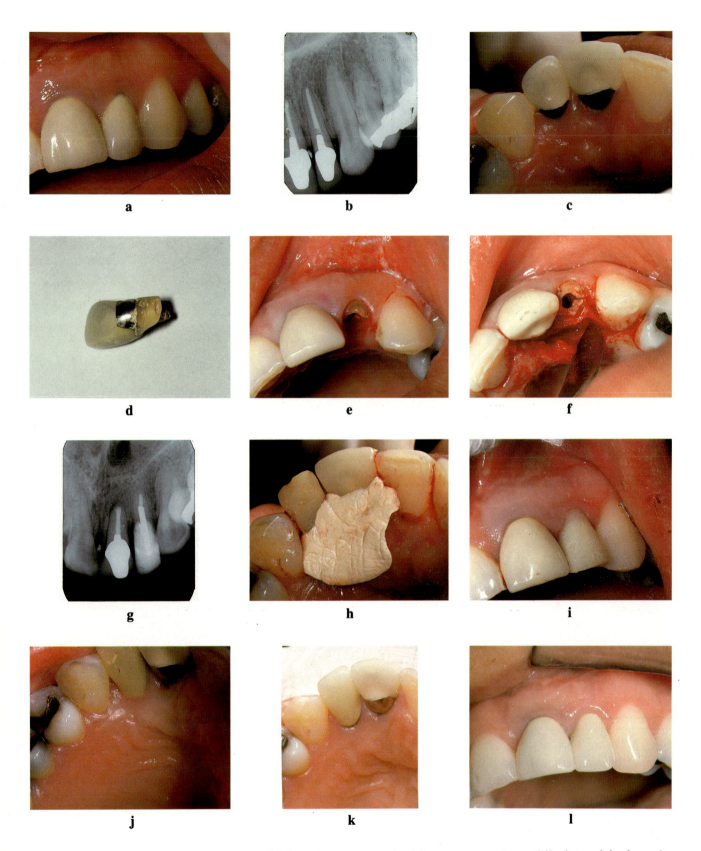

Fig. 3-26. a. The patient, a 25-year-old female, presented with an extremely mobile lateral incisor. **b.** Radiograph of the tooth. **c.** Lingual view. **d.** The tooth was anesthetized and the mobile (continued)

Fig. 3-26. (continued) portion removed, severing lingual gingival attachments. **e.** Fractured tooth from the labial. **f.** Lingual perspective showing ragged fracture extending several millimeters apical to the crestal bone level. **g.** The fracture was smoothed, lingual bone was recontoured to the fracture line, and soft tissue was excised to the bone level. When hemostasis was achieved, a post was cemented into the canal, a pin was inserted labially, and a composite buildup was placed 3 mm coronal to the lingual bone level. The new biologic width was created on a portion of fractured dentin. **h.** Pack in place over the lingual wound. **i.** Labial aspect of the provisional restoration (buildup). **j.** Lingual view of the restoration three months later. Shortly after this time, a new crown was inserted with the lingual margin just apical to the composite buildup. **k.** Postoperative healing one year later—lingual. **l.** Postoperative healing one year later—labial.

Case 3
Fracture of Mandibular First Molar

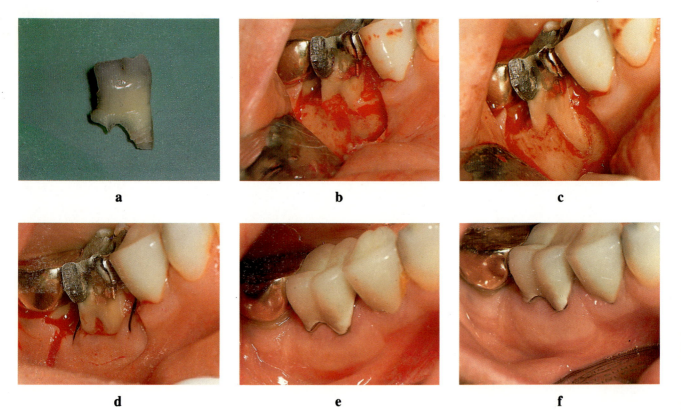

a   b   c

d   e   f

Fig. 3-27. a. This is the fractured buccal aspect of a crown from an endodontically treated tooth. **b.** Instead of extracting the tooth, the operator decided to attempt saving it. A full-thickness trapezoidal flap reflection reveals the damage. Sharp bone remains after the removal of fractured tooth structure. The fracture was 4-5 mm apical to the crestal bone level. **c.** Bone was smoothed with a round carbide bur to the level of the tooth fracture. **d.** The flap was repositioned at the bone level. **e.** Six-month postoperative picture. A new periodontal attachment has been formed with epithelial and connective tissue attachments on fractured dentine. This is a compromised, albeit healthy, result due to iatrogenic intervention. **f.** Three-year postoperative picture.

Case 4
Endodontically Treated, Severely Decayed Mandibular Bicuspid

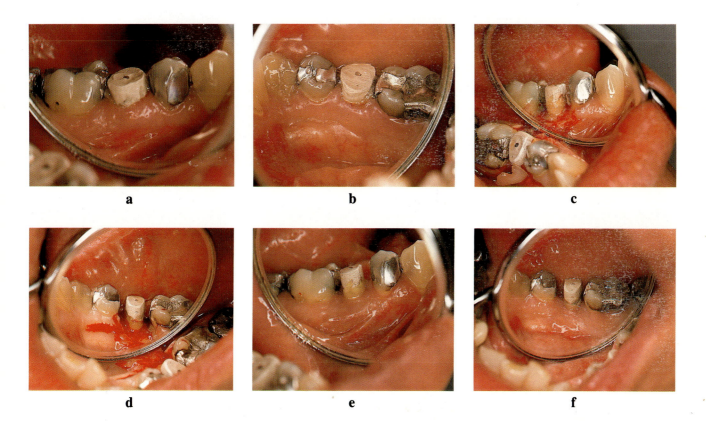

Fig. 3-28. a. This decayed, nonvital mandibular bicuspid was restored with a post/core buildup. **b.** Buildup margins are deeply subgingival on all sides and there is a short clinical crown. **c.** During crown lengthening surgery, a flap was reflected, followed by osseous recontouring on all surfaces. Releasing incisions help provide better access. Buccal view. **d.** Lingual view. **e.** Six weeks postoperatively, soft tissue is seen to be healing well and will continue to mature over the next 2-4 weeks. **f.** There now is 2-3 mm of sound tooth structure apical to the buildup margin, to use in completing the final restoration.

Case 5
Decayed Maxillary Lateral Incisor

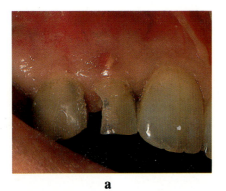
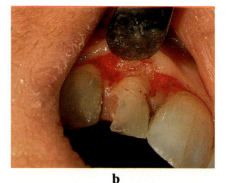

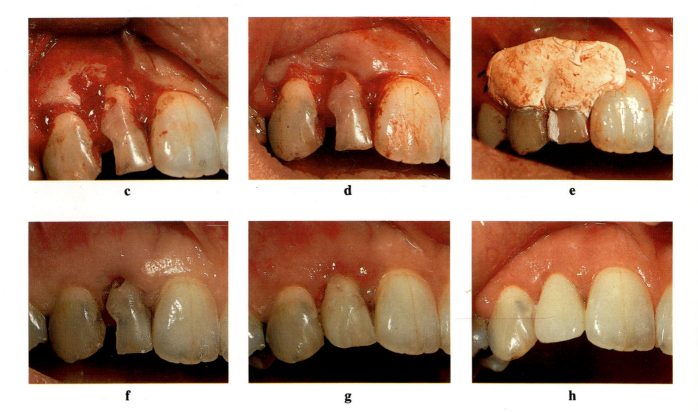

Fig. 3-29. a. This tooth has decay at the gingival level on the distal, it is endodontically involved, and there is a sinus tract stoma in labial-attached gingiva 3 mm from the free margin. **b.** This exploratory full-thickness flap was reflected to assess the nature of the pathology. Under the soft tissue lesion there is labial decay. **c.** The flap was enlarged and osseous remodeling was accomplished with a bur exposing close to 3 mm of labial bone. **d.** The flap was approximated apical to its original position to evaluate how healing might take place. **e.** A provisional (IRM) restoration was inserted, the flap was sutured, and periopack was placed over the flap. **f.** One month following surgery. The IRM was removed to allow for a post and composite buildup. **g.** Composite buildup in the tooth—day of placement. **h.** Two months later. Porcelain fused to metal crown shown on the day of insertion.

Case 6
Mandibular Canine and Bicuspid:
Short Crowns and Subgingival Canine Decay

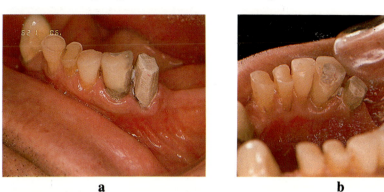

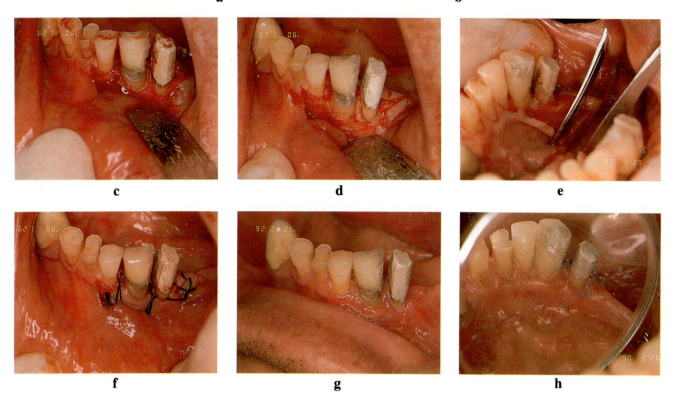

Fig. 3-30. a. These mandibular teeth (canine and bicuspid) have both been endodontically treated and restored with post/core buildups. On the canine, there is labial subgingival decay. **b.** Buildup margins on the bicuspid are subgingival on all surfaces. **c.** Flap reflection shows little tooth structure between the buildup material and the osseous crest. Restoration without crown lengthening would violate "biologic width." Flap reflection extends both mesially and distally approximately one additional tooth with mesial and distal releasing incisions. On the lingual there is only one releasing incision to the distal to provide greater visualization and access. **d.** After bone removal, there is at least 3 mm of root surface coronal to the osseous crest on all surfaces. Facial view. **e.** Lingual view. **f.** Flaps are positioned and sutured at the tooth/bone junction. **g.** At six weeks postoperatively, teeth are stable and soft tissues are healing well. There is at least a 2 mm band of sound tooth structure available supragingivally for the design and fabrication of a quality restoration. Facial view. **h.** Lingual view.

Case 7
Mandibular Canine with Crown Fractured Off Below the Gingival Level

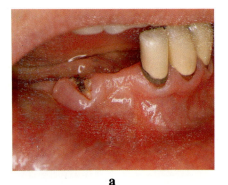

a

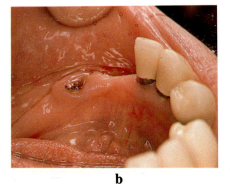

b

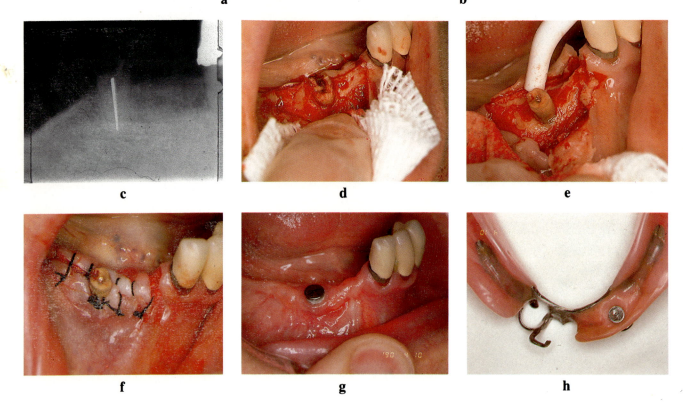

c   d   e

f   g   h

Fig. 3-31. a. The existing root stalk of this canine is decayed to the level of the osseous crest. It is the only abutment tooth on this side for a partial denture. Labial view. **b.** Lingual view. **c.** Radiographic view. **d.** The flap reflection extends mesially and distally with releasing incisions for good visibility. This access enables the operator to make a smooth, blended transition with osseous recontouring. A small flap would restrict the operator to an abrupt trough around the tooth. The tooth is severely decayed, at least to crestal bone. **e.** After decay removal and ostectomy, there is at least 3 mm of sound root for establishing "biologic width" and for physiologic margin placement. **f.** Flaps are apically repositioned and sutured. **g.** Soft tissue healing at 8 weeks postoperatively. Gingival health is good and there is adequate attached gingiva present. The tooth has been restored with a cemented post and magnetic keeper attachment. **h.** The magnet is retained inside the partial denture. Despite minimal periodontal support, the tooth is stable, comfortable, and provides excellent retention and stability for the partial denture appliance.

References

1. Maynard JG, and Wilson RD. Physiologic dimension of the periodontium to the restorative dentist. *J Periodont*. 1979;50:170.

2. Davis JW, et al. Periodontal surgery as an adjunct to endodontics, orthodontics, and restorative dentistry. *JADA*. 1987;115:271.

3. Kohavi D, and Stern N. Crown lengthening procedure Part II. Treatment planning and surgical considerations. *Comp of Cont Ed in Dent*. 1983;4(5):413.

Additional Reading Material

1. Pruthi VK. Surgical crown lengthening in periodontics. *J Canadian Dent Assn*. 1987;53(12):911.

2. Meister F, et al. Periodontal considerations in clinical crown lengthening procedures. *Gen Dent*. 1981;29(5):401.

3. Ingber JS, Rose IF, and Coslet JC. The "biologic width"—a concept in periodontics and restorative dentistry. *Alpha Omegan*. 1977;70:62.

4. Kohavi D, and Stern N. Crown lengthening procedure, Part I. Clinical aspects. *Comp of Cont Ed in Dent*. 1983;4(4):347.

5. Allen EP. Periodontic support for the restorative dentist. *Texas Dental Journal*. 1984;101(11):32.

Chapter 4

Apicoectomy and Retroseal Techniques For Anterior Teeth

INTRODUCTION

Cleansing a root canal and sealing it from the periodontal ligament and surrounding bone usually ensures health of the attachment apparatus. Necrotic canals give rise to protein degradation products, bacteria, and bacterial toxins that can result in periapical pathology. Voids at the apex cause stagnation of tissue fluids, leading to periapical percolation and irritation. These problems are avoided by using proper root canal instrumentation, disinfection, and obturation.

Endodontic therapy is generally accomplished by conservative means with coronal access. When performed in this manner the success rate is near 90 percent.[1-4] However, what if there is failure of conventional endodontic treatment? How should it be managed? Some see a controversy between the nonsurgical and the surgical approach to retreatment of these failures. Actually, there is no controversy. Such arguments are eliminated by understanding the cause of failure and what is to be accomplished by retreatment. If nonsurgical retreatment is feasible, it should be attempted. Dental literature shows that the success of retreatment is higher when done nonsurgically and that the success of surgery is higher when it follows nonsurgical retreatment.[4] The ultimate purpose of surgery is to establish a lasting seal that will not be subject to the future percolation of fluids in and out of the canal.[5]

One way to classify nonsurgical retreatment is by the type of filling material that is being removed from the involved canal, i.e., gutta-percha, pastes, silver points, and so forth. Some are easier to remove than others. Often the initial treatment renders the case compromised by iatrogenic factors. Some operator-caused failures are from broken instruments, ledged canals, perforated chambers, floors and roots, and unretrievable fillings. Occasionally, failure is from anatomic factors over which an operator has little or no control, such as lateral or calcified canals. Prior to either conventional retreatment or surgery, one should review the history of previous treatment, take x-rays at different angles and compare them, check for occlusal trauma, evaluate the vitality and general condition of adjacent teeth, and examine sulci for periodontal pockets or evidence of vertical fractures.

CASE SELECTION

The table below presents a list of indications that suggest the need to perform periapical surgery.

Table 4-1. Possible Indications for Endodontic Surgery

Anatomic Complications of the Root Canal System
- calcified canals
- impassable pulp stones (denticles)
- severely curved canals
- non-negotiable apical development
- incomplete apical development
- root resorption
- the fenestration of root apices through the cortical plate

Iatrogenic Problems
- non-soluble material in the root canal
- irretrievable filling materials
- post and cores
- impassable ledges
- perforations
- over-instrumentation (vertical)
- gross overfills
- persistent pre-obturation pain
- persistent post-obturation pain

Known Trauma
- horizontal root fracture near the apex with pulpal necrosis
- avulsion

Expediency of Treatment
- relief of pain or swelling
- inability to disinfect the canal or control exudate
- insufficient time to wait for normal healing

Unusual History of Lesion
- grown very fast
- caused extensive bone destruction

Failure of Previous Endodontics/Diagnostic Considerations
- no apparent cause—filling and seal appear adequate
- cause may become evident during surgery

Levels of Surgical Difficulty

There are three levels of surgical difficulty for apicoectomy and retroseal procedures. The first level is well within the scope of most general practitioners. Whether or not generalists perform cases within levels two and three depends on interest in surgery, experience, and their general "comfort zone."

Table 4-2. Levels of Surgical Difficulty with Endodontic Surgery (from least to greatest difficulty)*

Level 1

Maxillary Central
Maxillary Lateral
Maxillary Canine

Level 2

Maxillary First Molar, Buccal Roots
Mandibular Central
Mandibular Lateral
Mandibular Canine
Maxillary First Premolar
Maxillary Second Premolar

Level 3

Maxillary Second Molar, Buccal Roots
Maxillary Molars, Palatal Roots
Mandibular Premolars
Mandibular Molars

* This breakdown is a generalization. There are some anatomic variations that would create exceptions.

Anatomy

In the maxilla, the alveolar process is closely approximated to the floor of the nose. If, coincidentally, a person has both a short alveolar process and long roots, the incisor apices may contact the thin bony plate of the nasal floor (Fig. 4-1a). This is especially true if the teeth are more vertically instead of labially inclined. Surgically, this is usually not a problem since during the apicoectomy procedure the root is going to be shortened and beveled anyway. Centrals are the main offenders.

Maxillary and mandibular canines and incisors often lack an adequate covering of labial cortical plate (Fig. 4-1, a-d). This can complicate the surgical procedure if certain precautions are not taken during flap design and reflection. Incisions made directly over thin bone or over bare, prominent roots can leave a bothersome fenestration in soft tissue postoperatively.

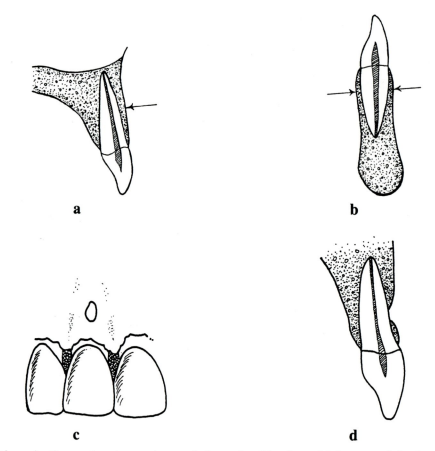

Fig. 4-1. Variations in Bony Anatomy Around Anterior Teeth **a,** This central incisor is supported only by thin bone labially and apically. Sometimes the floor of the nose is in fairly close proximity to the end of the root as depicted here. The main precaution in this case is to exercise care in debridement. **b,** This lower incisor has thin bone labially and lingually. **c,** When thin labial bone is combined with a prominent root as seen in this illustration, a bony fenestration may result. **d,** Lateral view of the fenestration shown in c. This anatomic situation contraindicates use of the semilunar flap design.

Some practitioners claim that periodontal defects such as marginal bone loss impair the prognosis of this procedure. Skoglund,[6] on the other hand, maintains that we should not rule out endodontic surgery on teeth with moderate periodontal disease, including deep periodontal pockets. He suggests that it should be performed, especially if the alternative is an otherwise unnecessary prosthetic reconstruction.

Maxillary canines, premolars, and first molars may have roots in close proximity to the maxillary sinus. Lesion curettage should be carefully done to prevent unnecessary laceration and penetration of the membrane. Sinus perforation is generally not a serious concern, but contamination and irritation with medications or filling material should be meticulously avoided. The reason the operator need not be alarmed about a communication into the sinus is that primary closure is easily obtained at the conclusion of the procedure, thus sealing the wound and facilitating normal healing. As with any sinus exposure, however, the normal triad of medications should routinely be given, namely, an antibiotic, a decongestant, and a nasal spray to help shrink the membrane.

The patient should always be notified of sinus proximity during the procedure and warned to avoid actions that would cause complications. Even the slightest membrane exposure could predispose rupture and even lead to air emphysema in the midface region from coughing, sneezing, or blowing the nose.

Mandibular incisors and canines may present difficult access during surgery because of their angulation and because of frequent shallow vestibular depth (high muscle attachments). The more labially inclined the crowns, the more lingually inclined will be their roots, thus complicating the procedure. In addition, lower canines may be "bow shaped" — convex in the labial mid-root region yet with an apex to the lingual and deep in the bone.

The size of the periapical lesion also has a bearing on potential difficulty. Generally, the larger the lesion (within reason) the easier the case. When there is no lesion, it is often hard to localize and identify the root for manipulation. Conversely, if the lesion is too large, even encompassing apices of adjacent teeth, this can complicate surgery, with the iatrogenic devitalization of teeth that would probably otherwise have remained healthy.

One reason for endodontic failure is the presence of one or more accessory canals in a given root. Green[7] localized one or more accessory canals to the apical 2.2 mm of 10 percent of anterior teeth. Ingle has summarized the anatomical characteristics of anterior teeth as follows:

Table 4-3. Selected Anatomical Characteristics of Anterior Teeth
(Adapted from Ingle JI and Taintor JF. *Endodontics*, 3rd ed. Philadelphia, Lee & Febiger, 1985.)

Teeth	Average Length	Lateral Canals	Number of Canals
Maxillary Centrals	23.2 mm	23%	1 canal 100%
Maxillary Laterals	22.8 mm	10%	1 canal 99.9%
Maxillary Canines	26.0 mm	24%	1 canal 100%
Mandibular Centrals	21.5 mm	5.2%	1 canal, 1 foramen 70.1% 2 canals, 1 foramen 23.4% 2 canals, 2 foramina 6.5%
Mandibular Laterals	22.4 mm	13.9%	1 canal, 1 foramen 56.9% 2 canals, 1 foramen 14.7% 2 canals, 2 foramina 29.4%
Mandibular Canines	25.2 mm	9.5%	1 canal, 94% 2 canals, 2 foramina 6%

Even though this chapter has narrowed its emphasis to only anterior teeth, some mention will be made of maxillary first molars. A recent clinical investigation by Neaverth, et al[8] reported that 77 percent of the mesiobuccal roots of these teeth had two canals.

Neaverth's study depicted a typical type of root canal system found in the mesiobuccal root of maxillary molars as having two main canals with numerous branching accessory canals (Fig. 4-2).

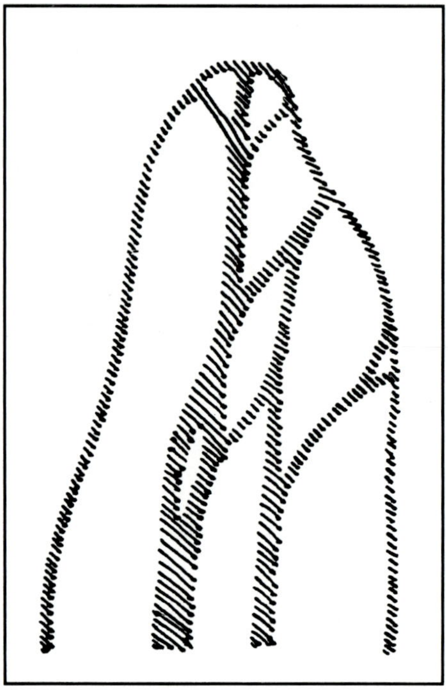

Fig. 4-2. Maxillary First Molar Mesiobuccal Root System. (Adapted from Neaverth EJ, Kotley LM, Kaltenbach RF. Clinical Investigation (in vivo) of endodontically treated maxillary first molars. *J Endodontics*. 1987;13(10):505-512.)

Patient Acceptance and Informed Consent

The high incidence of anomalous canals is a primary reason why we will continue to have treatment failures with conventional endodontic therapy, despite the best possible treatment by practitioners. Dentists should be wary of creating unrealistic expectations in the minds of patients regarding the anticipated outcome of treatment. Many dentists are now using consent forms with endodontics (*see Tables 4-4 and 4-5*). In some states, this area of dental practice is the leading cause of professional liability claims.

Practitioners and patients must also be aware that periapical surgery is not a cure-all for endodontic problems. Just as conventional endodontics is only about 90 percent successful in the hands of good operators, surgical endodontics will resolve symptoms only about 90 percent of the time. If this fact is not communicated adequately to the patient, it could spawn subsequent medicolegal difficulties.

Table 4-4. Sample of a consent form some dentists use prior to conventional endodontic treatment.

CONSENT FOR ROOT CANAL THERAPY   Tooth # _____

1. Root canal therapy is about 90-95 percent successful. Many factors influence a patient's individual healing: general health, adequate gum attachment and bone support, shape and condition of the roots and nerve canals, quality of previous dental care, pre-existing root fracture, etc.

2. Teeth treated with root canals must be protected during treatment. Between appointments, your tooth will have a temporary cement filling. If this should come out, please call the office and arrange to have it replaced.

3. Teeth treated with root canals can still decay, but since the nerve is gone, there will be no pain. As with other teeth, the proper care of these teeth consists of good home care, a sensible diet, and periodic dental check-ups.

4. The tooth may be sensitive after appointments and even remain tender for a period of time after treatment has been finished. If sensitivity persists and does not seem to be getting better (even a few weeks after the root canal has been completed) please call the office.

5. In some teeth, regular root canal therapy alone may not be sufficient. For example, if the canals are severely bent or calcified, if there is substantial infection in the bone around the roots, or if a file becomes segmented within a canal, the tooth may remain sensitive and an oral surgery procedure may be necessary to resolve the problem.

6. Root fracture is one of the main reasons why root canals fail. Unfortunately, some cracks that extend from the crown down into the root are invisible and undetectable. They can occur on uncrowned teeth from traumatic injury, biting on hard objects, habitual clenching or grinding, and even just normal wear and tear. Whether the fracture occurs before or after the root canal, it will probably still require extraction.

7. Teeth treated with root canals will be more brittle than other teeth, and subject to cracks or fractures. After the root canal, the tooth could possibly be filled with either a silver or a tooth-colored filling. However, to prevent damage that might mean losing the tooth, crowning (capping) is the best treatment. This is especially important with molar and bicuspid teeth.

8. There are alternatives to root canal therapy. They include no treatment at all; extraction; and extraction followed by a bridge, partial denture, or implant.

The nature of root canal therapy has been explained to me and I have had an opportunity to have any questions answered. I understand that dentistry is not an exact science and success with root canals cannot be guaranteed. If a case is beyond a certain level of complexity, the doctor will suggest that I be referred to a specialist to have the work done. In light of the above information, I hereby authorize _____ to proceed with treatment.

_____   _____
Patient Name (please print)   Date

_____
Signature (guardian if patient is a minor)

Table 4-5. Sample of a generic consent form some dentists use prior to surgical endodontic treatment.

Patient's Name: _____   Date: _____

Doctor's Name: _____   Phone: _____

    INFORMED CONSENT: The dental treatment necessary to my existing oral condition(s) has been explained to me and my questions have been answered satisfactorily. I hereby authorize _____ and/or associates or assistants as he may designate to perform those procedures, including surgery, as may be deemed necessary or advisable for my dental treatment, including arrangement and/or administration of any anesthetic, sedative, analgesic, therapeutic and/or other sedative, analgesic, medicinal or drug treatment(s) and do voluntarily assume any or all possible risks which may be associated with these procedures and/or with any of the following procedures:

_____

_____

_____

_____

_____

Signature: _____   Date: _____
      (patient or legal guardian of patient)

Witness: _____

Possible Referral Criteria

    Referral of a case by a generalist to a specialist will depend on several factors. It most frequently involves overall difficulty coupled with the operator's experience and existing "comfort zone." Some of the factors that might•require greater than normal expertise (referral) are listed below.

1. No radiolucency or periapical bony defect present. Sometimes it is difficult to differentiate tooth from bone when they are immediately contiguous.
2. Defect too large. This may involve roots of other teeth with the potential for devitalization.
3. Anatomical considerations:
    a. Tooth root angulated to the lingual, limiting access and visibility.
    b. Very shallow mucobuccal fold necessitating extensive soft tissue reflection (mainly occurs in the lower arch).
    c. Short alveolar ridges and long roots.
    d. Very prominent tooth with suspected lack of bone on labial.
4. Periodontal pathology
    a. Periodontitis with questionable prognosis.
5. Need for special patient management

Surgical Treatment

A list of instruments and supplies for endodontic surgery are listed in Table 4-6.

Table 4-6. Instruments and Supplies Used With Endodontic Surgery

1. Dental mirror
2. Cotton plier
3. Syringe, needle, and local anesthetic (Xylocaine 2%. 1:50,000)
4. Irrigation syringe (such as Monoject 412) and saline
5. Fine suction tip
6. Scalpel and #15 blade
7. Periosteal elevator such as the Molt #9
8. Wide flap retractor such as the Seldin 23, Minnesota, or HF #1 single-ended retractor
9. Periodontal curette
10. Surgical (spoon) curette
11. Endodontic explorer
12. Regular dental explorer
13. Metal ruler
14. Needle holder
15. Surgical scissors
16. Suture material
17. Autoclavable handpieces for root resection and retropreparation
    - high-speed (that does not force air into the surgical field) or straight handpiece
    - micro contra-angle for straight handpiece (Fig. 4-3) *(The microhead handpiece with short microburs demands only 10 mm clearance apical to the root, thus facilitating a perpendicular entry.)*
18. Carbide burs (as needed)
    - 701 or 702 fissure for straight handpiece
    - small round or inverted cones for microhead
19. Carrier for restorative material
    - regular amalgam carrier (small end)
    - mini amalgam carriers (such as the K-G retrofilling amalgam carrier, Fig. 4-3)
20. Amalgam plugger
21. 2x2 gauze
22. Sterile gauze (cotton pellets are in disfavor because of residual fibers left behind)
23. Bone wax (optional)

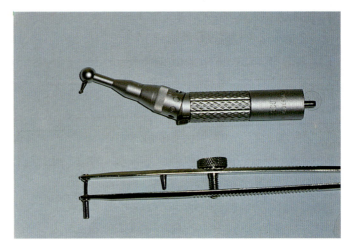

Fig. 4-3. Microhead Handpiece and Micro Amalgam Carrier.

THE SURGICAL PROCEDURE

Flap Designs

In this chapter, four different flap designs are presented for use with periapical surgery. They are **triangular**, **trapezoidal**, **semilunar** and **modified semilunar**.

General Considerations in Flap Design

Prior to the incisions, the patient should be instructed to bite on a folded 2x2 gauze pad. This helps the individual maintain a comfortable jaw position throughout the procedure. Gauze can also be placed laterally on both sides of the surgical site to help control bleeding.

A flap should be chosen which provides good access for visibility and instrumentation without causing unnecessary irritation to the tissues. After the procedure, this flap is repositioned to protect the wound and promote healing. Full-thickness mucoperiosteal flaps are incised, reflected, and retracted with sharp instruments to minimize tissue damage.

Factors that help determine flap selection

Anatomical

- height and depth of the vestibule
- root eminences
- frenum size, shape, and location
- nature of the soft tissue
- sulcus depth
- smile line (amount of gingiva showing when smiling)

Esthetic

- crowns with subgingival margins

Periodontal

- labial and interproximal pocket formation
- gingival recession

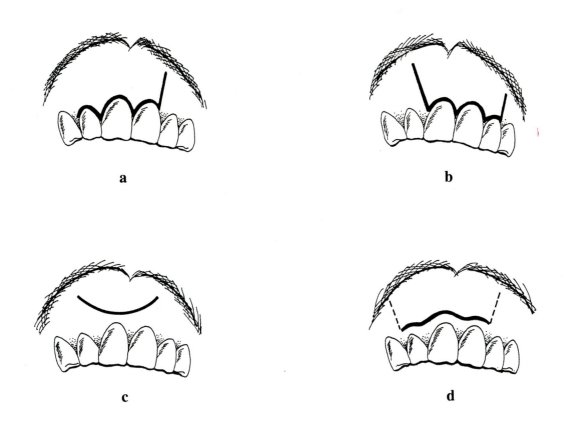

Fig. 4-4. Illustrations of Recommended Flap Designs **a, Triangular or three-cornered flap.** Releasing incisions are generally made at an oblique angle to the horizontal portion to preserve the blood supply at their juncture. **b, Trapezoidal flap.** If neighboring teeth have prominent roots and labial bone is suspected to be thin or missing, releasing segments prevent postoperative healing problems such as dehiscences along the incision line. **c, Semilunar flap. d, Modified semilunar flap.** With the horizontal portion in attached gingiva and without the releasing segments, this is sometimes termed an "attached gingiva" flap.

Discussion of Various Flap Options and Characteristics of Each

Triangular Flap

- With any releasing-type incision that crosses a prominent root, postoperative soft tissue fenestrations or dehiscences may occur in cases where there is:

    a) no bone or thin bone beneath the mucosa

    b) a poor blood supply

- These areas, which usually present as root prominences, should not have incisions made over them. Rather, incisions should be made in the troughs between the roots.

- Releasing incisions

    a) Must be long enough to prevent pulling and overmanipulation

    b) Should not vertically bisect the papillae

    c) Should contact a tooth at its line angle

- A disadvantage with reflecting gingiva along the gingival margin (triangular and trapezoidal flaps) is that it can cause gingival recession due to crestal bone resorption and remodeling.[5] This, in turn, may expose the margin of a crown or veneer that previously was covered with tissue.

Trapezoidal Flap

- Provides greater access and visibility and less tissue tension than a triangular flap.
- Involves two vertical or oblique incisions, each made at least one full tooth to the side of the involved tooth.
- Preferable to include papillae, if present, and not cut laterally across them.
- In deference to supplying adequate vasculature, the base must always be wider than the coronal edge.
- Gives a good view of periodontal defects and bony fenestrations.
- Will allow periodontal surgery to be performed as part of the operation.
- Heals with minimum scar tissue.
- Preferred over some other designs when handling the frenum (cutting horizontally through the frenum makes it hard to keep the incision "in-line" which delays healing and predisposes scarring).
- Often preferred with shallow vestibules where it is sometimes hard to get adequate reflection (in those cases, it is usually helpful if the releasing segments are more obliquely flared).

Semilunar Flap

- Formerly the most common flap design (replaced by the modified semilunar).
- Maintains attached and marginal gingiva intact.
- The curved, convex portion should be in attached gingiva.
- Needs lateral extension for good access (extending at least one tooth on either side of the one involved).
- The apogee of the curve (nearest the teeth) should be at least 1 mm apical to the depth of the gingival sulcus or about 5 mm from the free margin. If it is made too close to the free marginal gingiva, then this thin isthmus of tissue may degenerate and begin to dehisce at the neck of the tooth.
- The incision must be made well outside the expected bone cavity on solid bone—preferably 4-5 mm from the bony defect. If too close to the osseous wound site, there is a greater chance of incision breakdown and delayed healing.
- If used in frenum area, should jog around this attachment.
- Used when there is no gingival recession or periodontal pocket.
- No sutures into the narrow band (isthmus) of gingiva near the crown of the tooth since even this minor compromise of tissue integrity may cause it to degenerate and dehisce. Suture on the more lateral aspects of the flap.

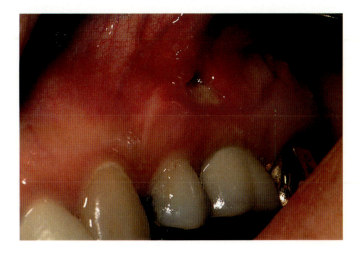

Fig. 4-5. Soft tissue fenestration and bone exposure from flap margin not having underlying bony support.

Modified Semilunar or Attached Gingiva Flap

- Has become a popular choice among endodontists.[3]

- Access is nearly as good as with the triangular flap.

- No disruption of marginal gingiva or interdental papillae.

- Horizontal component in attached gingiva and at least 1 mm apical to the depth of the gingival sulcus (usually 5 mm apical to the free gingival margin).

- Contraindicated when there are labial periodontal pockets or gingival recession. In such cases, use a triangular or trapezoidal flap design instead.

- Easy to reposition and results in little scarring.

- Suture into papillae.

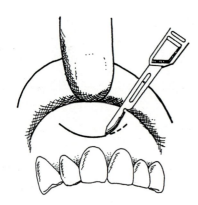

1.

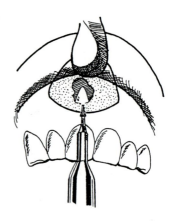

2.

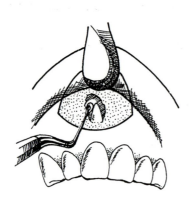

3.

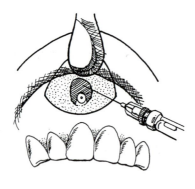

4.

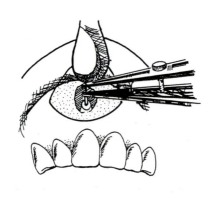

5.

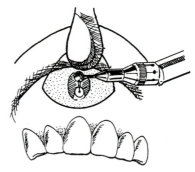

6.

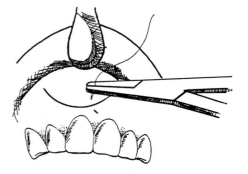

7.

8.

Fig. 4-6. Sequence of steps required for surgery

Figure 4-6 shows a step-by-step progression for periapical surgery.

1. The scalpel handle is held in a pen grasp to make the desired incision. A #15 blade is being used.

2. A periodontal curette is applied to determine the density of the cortical plate. If bone is perforated, it may be removed with the curette or with a bur.

3. Granulation tissue is removed with either the periodontal curette or, as seen here, a surgical spoon curette.

4. A bur is used to enlarge the opening (if necessary), to resect the apical 2 mm of the root, and to bevel the root at a 45° angle. This step makes the lingual part of the defect even more accessible to debridement.

5. If periapical bone is sensitive, anesthetic can be injected into bone under pressure. This also aids hemostasis.

6. The microhead handpiece is shown creating a 2 mm deep retropreparation at the apex in the long axis of the root.

7. After good hemostasis is achieved both from soft tissue and bone, the filling material is carried to the root and condensed into the retropreparation. Here a K-G retrofilling amalgam carrier was selected.

8. Sutures are placed toward the interproximal areas where there is more attached gingiva. Try to avoid the thin "isthmus" of tissue on the labial of the root.

Exposure of the Surgical Site

Incisions

Incisions for a particular case will conform to the flap design selected. Each component should be made in a single stroke with a sharp scalpel, and should not be choppy or jagged.

Flap reflection

Mucoperiosteal flaps are full-thickness reflections. If the pathologic material has penetrated cortical bone and adheres to the periosteum, then it should be disengaged by blunt or sharp dissection. Excision of a fistulous tract in the mucosa is not necessary.

Flap retraction

Retraction of the flap is a passive measure. The retractor rests carefully on bone. It must be wide enough to give good visibility and not allow soft tissue to sag around the instrument into the proximity of the bur.

Osteotomy

Bone overlying the periapical defect should be "tested" with a periodontal curette or other suitable instrument to evaluate its soundness and integrity. If intact, the labial cortical plate over the root apex is usually removed with a bur, although in some cases a rongeur may be used. The root apex is localized by measuring from the tooth's incisal edge to the apex with a sterile metal ruler. This distance is obtained from x-rays or measurements from previous endodontic treatment. One rule of thumb is that the root length is generally one and one-half crown lengths. Still another localization method is to start a cut in the bone, place a small piece of metal over what is thought to be the apical area and take an x-ray to help pinpoint the exact spot. Bone removal should give good access to the root tip and the periapical lesion.

Curettage and Biopsy

Granulomatous tissue is removed from the bony defect with a curette (periodontal or surgical spoon). If a defect is so large that it involves the apices of adjacent teeth, the operator must be careful to avoid their devitalization. Kruger[9] mentions that all cystic or granulomatous material at the apex need not be removed if it might endanger the health of an adjacent tooth. Generally 20% or so can be left without adverse sequelae.

If a cyst is present the operator should try to accomplish enucleation by placing a spoon curette between the cyst lining and the bony wall. At the initial stage of enucleation, the convex side of the instrument should be placed against the cyst lining. Periapical tissue should be placed in a specimen bottle containing formalin and submitted to an oral pathologist for histologic examination.[10]

Lesions of maxillary anteriors that erode palatal bone heal following surgery, but **radiographically they may always appear to have a periapical lesion at the apex.** This is because of residual scarring. The patient should be made aware of this phenomenon.

Apicoectomy

An apicoectomy is performed by resecting the most apical portion of the root. Since studies reveal one or more accessory canals in the apical two millimeters or so of 10% of anterior teeth, it follows that the tip should be removed to this extent (about 2 mm). Most dentists use a 701, 702, or a round bur (lessens sharp line angles). Some are also using lasers.[11] The root is beveled from the labial so that the freshly cut end of the root is visible from the labial.

Following this apical resection, *maxillary* roots are cut at about a 45-degree angle, whereas the desired angle with *mandibular* incisors is somewhat greater than 45 degrees. It is more acute with lower teeth because the eye level is above the apex and one's line of vision is directed downward. Increasing the angle provides better visibility and access.

Reasons for removing the root apex

1. Unfilled apical branches of the main root canal, which may have been invaded by micro-organisms, are eliminated.
2. Access is achieved by which to seal the root canal.
3. Access to diseased tissue lingual to the root is improved.[12]

Root end resections of well-condensed gutta-percha/sealer obturations do not adversely affect a seal, but resections of silver points do.[13]

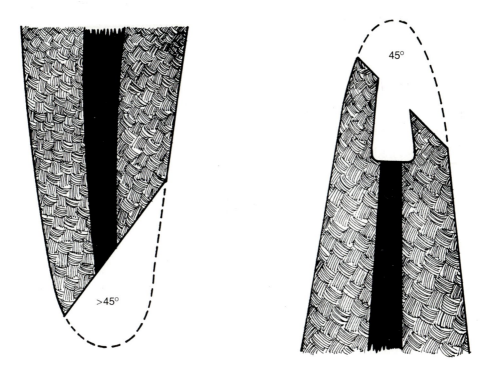

Mandibular   **Maxillary**

Fig. 4-7. Apicoectomy Angulations for Anterior Teeth. Mandibular roots are often beveled at an angle greater than 45 degrees to enhance visibility of the root apex and access for instrumentation. Maxillary roots are generally beveled at a 45-degree angle.

Root apices protruding through cortical bone:

Bony fenestrations and protruding roots palpable through mucosa are asymptomatic when the pulp is vital, but they can present with vague symptoms following conventional endodontic therapy or periapical surgery. The solution to the problem is a beveled resection of the apex to position it back within its bony housing.[3]

Retropreparation

Prior to cutting a preparation into the apex, the hollow area around the root is packed (with unfilled sterile gauze, bone wax, iodoform gauze, etc.) to minimize bleeding and help to collect displaced fragments of the filling material.[14] *Cotton packing is not recommended* since residual fibers left in the wound can cause delayed healing and a postoperative foreign body reaction. The packing material is removed from the defect prior to suturing. If bleeding persists, several options are available to achieve hemostasis. Among them are:

- **Xylocaine** with 1:50,000 epinephrine. Inject into soft tissue or bone as needed.

- **Bone wax**. This can be placed prior to making the retropreparation so that it does not enter the preparation and inadvertently prevent an apical seal. If used after the preparation is complete, gauze should be placed in the apex to prevent contamination. The soft wax is placed into the bony defect and then removed (as much as possible) prior to closure.

- **Electrocautery of soft tissue**.
- **Other recommendations** for controlling hemorrhage are:
  - crushing bleeding points
  - pressure with gauze
  - gauze moistened with a hemostatic agent

If the sinus is exposed (more common with canines than incisors), a gauze net should be used to prevent contaminants such as bone wax or filling materials from unwanted entry.

Traditional preparation in the long axis of the tooth

The apical foramen is located with an explorer. Once it is found, an appropriate handpiece and bur can be used to make the preparation. The micro contra-angle handpiece is preferred. Depending on access requirements, a conventional high-speed handpiece or slow-speed contra-angle could also be used.

Bur sizes and types are recommended below:

- Small root apex — 1/2 to 1 round bur
- Larger apex — 2 or 4 round bur
- To undercut the preparation: 33 1/2 or 35 inverted cone

Barry[15] recommends cutting the preparation to a depth of 2 mm. This is in general agreement with most major authors, although Arens[1] suggests the depth should be at least 3 mm. It should be kept small but include the entire foramen outline, have a well-defined shape, and be in the long axis of the root to the extent that is possible. An undercut is advised, but lateral overpreparation should be avoided to prevent weakening or perforation of the root. Kruger[9] recommends that because of there being more dentin on the lingual aspect of the tooth, the undercut only be made on that side of the prep. Because there is some dimensional instability with amalgam, roots can eventually split if the cross section ratio of amalgam to tooth is too great. This is especially the case if a low copper alloy containing zinc is used in the presence of moisture.

The "slot" retropreparation:

There are instances, such as with lower incisors, when one may choose to use a special kind of preparation such as a slot or Matsura type retropreparation. Its indications are:

1. Limited access
2. Extreme lingual tipping
3. Minimal root structure to be removed.

The method has disadvantages. These include:

1. Harder to see and debride the lingual aspect of the defect
2. More extensive intracanal preparation
3. More filling material in contact with tissues.

The technique is as follows (Fig. 4-8.):

- The root is beveled labially.
- A 5 mm long slot is prepared with a fine fissure bur that extends into the canal.
- An inverted cone or round bur is used inside the slot to establish a dovetail or retentive lock.
- The filling material can be condensed from the labial rather than only from the apex.

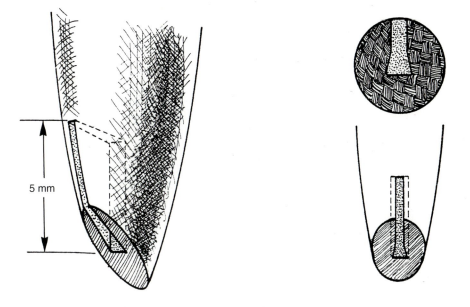

Fig. 4-8. Slot Preparation. A slot is cut into the apex extending from the outer root surface straight into the canal. It is approximately 5 mm in vertical height and as wide as the bur being used (about 1mm). At its depth, the slot may be undercut slightly (creating a dovetail) to assist with retention of the filling material. The cross-sectional view shows the inner dovetail created by undercutting.

Retroseal

Upon completion of the retropreparation the field is dried and a restoration is inserted. A good retrosealing material will have the following properties:

- well-tolerated
- provides a tight seal
- easy to manipulate and condense
- radiopaque
- bacteriostatic (or at least not encouraging bacterial growth)
- dimensionally stable
- impervious to moisture
- fast setting time
- not easily dislodged
- not carcinogenic

Amalgam

The material most commonly used in the past has been a high-copper containing spherical alloy. Zinc-free amalgam is preferred since there is less expansion in the event it is contaminated with moisture. A low-copper zinc containing alloy contaminated with moisture could exhibit delayed expansion of a magnitude to induce root fracture.[16]

Amalgam is recommended by Tronstad,[17] Birn and Winther,[18] Laskin,[19] Burke,[2] Grossman,[20] Bramwell,[21] Barry,[22] and Ingle.[3] It is used even though it may have such disadvantages as corrosion, introduction of mercury into periapical tissues, amalgam particle scattering, and some leakage. Before condensing the restoration, the preparation should be lined with cavity varnish.[12,17,23] The amalgam must be placed securely, since if dislodged, it can act as a foreign body and adversely affect prior treatment.[24]

Laskin[19] suggests that it is desirable to have a slight concavity in the amalgam restoration to avoid a flash at the margin. Excess amalgam should be carefully removed from the surgical site (bone and soft tissue) to prevent the metallic "shotgun" appearance on the postoperative radiograph. *See Figure 4-9.*

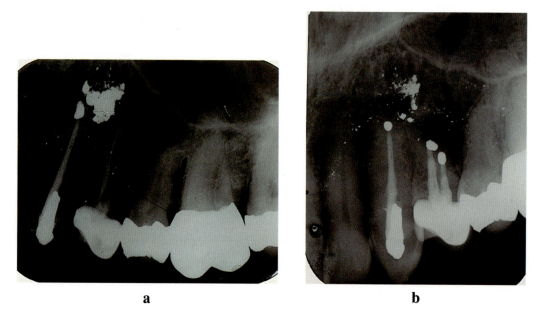

a   b

Fig. 4-9. a. There is massive amalgam scatter following an apicoectomy and retroseal procedure. **b.** This view follows an endodontist's attempt to clean up the area.

Amalgam alternatives

Amalgam alternatives listed in recent dental literature include IRM and EBA cement,[25,26] glass ionomer cement,[12,27-29] gold foil,[30] injectable gutta-percha,[31-32] conventional gutta-percha,[33] and bone cement.[34] Older research has suggested such materials as Cavit (polyvinyl zinc oxide cement), zinc phosphate cement, Adaptic, poly-HEMA (methyl acrylate), and Durelon (polycarboxylate cement).

Based on findings in existing dental literature, the author recommends IRM and SuperEBA cement as strong choices for materials to use in place of the the traditional "amalgam."

Filling material for conventional endodontics

Gutta-percha is the most common filling material for conventional endodontic therapy. Most endodontists believe that although paste fillings are initially successful, they have too great a capacity for resorption. Silver points lack the necessary adaptability to the canal wall to provide a proper seal. For conventional endodontics, gutta-percha with sealer is the material of choice since it can be condensed to provide a hermetic seal.

Why retropreparation and retroseal following laterally condensed gutta-percha procedure? Why not just do an apicoectomy and burnish with a warm instrument?

- Some of the filling material may stick to the hot instrument and be teased away during the "sealing" process.
- Warm, burnished gutta-percha may recede from canal walls upon cooling.[15]
- Marginal defects produced by heat burnishing gutta-percha are ten times greater than defects existing with an amalgam fill. If burnishing is done at all, cold burnishing is far better than heat burnishing.[35]

Closure

The following ideas are helpful in the completion of the surgical part of the case:

1. Always take an x-ray prior to suturing.[14] This film will:
    - insure cleanliness,
    - check the level of the root amputation, and
    - serve as a reference for future healing.
2. Pathological tissue is submitted to a lab for histological examination.
3. Press on the flap for a minute or two before suturing to gain initial adherence.
4. Place interrupted sutures 2-3 mm from incision line (they hold better in attached gingiva.)
5. Do not suture too tightly.
6. Keep knots away from the incision line.

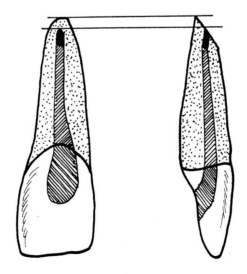

Radiographic View   **Anatomic Cross Section**

Fig. 4-10. Evaluation of the Retrofill on a Radiograph. The filling will appear short of the apex because of the diagonal nature of the cut and the fact that lingual tooth structure extends apical to the filling material.

Follow-up Care

What should the patient expect following the procedure?

1. Moderate pain that can be controlled with nonsteroidal anti-inflammatory (NSAI) agents or narcotic analgesics
2. Swelling for a few days
3. Possibly ecchymosis for 3-7 days
4. A temporary loss of feeling in the operated area
5. Some mobility of the affected tooth

Postoperative instructions are given in Table 4-7.

Table 4-7. An example of postoperative instructions given to patients.

Postoperative Instructions

1. By following these instructions you will play an important role in aiding the healing process and maintaining comfort.

2. Maintain gentle pressure for at least 10 minutes on the gauze sponge that has been placed over the surgical site. A slight oozing of blood from the area is normal for a few hours. If unusual bleeding occurs or a jelly-like clot forms, gently wipe the area with a damp gauze sponge, replace with another sponge, and hold under firm pressure until bleeding stops. A slightly dampened tea bag is very effective in controlling more profuse bleeding. If bleeding is not controlled, call this office.

3. Swelling and discoloration are normal following any surgical procedure. These problems can be minimized by the use of an ice pack, rest, and the avoidance of strenuous activities for the remainder of the day. Place the ice pack on your face, over the surgical area, for 10 minutes on and 5 minutes off. Alternate these intervals for up to 5-6 hours. It is advisable to elevate your head with pillows while sleeping to reduce pressure and potential bleeding.

4. Avoid mouth rinses today, as they stimulate bleeding. Gentle rinsing every 3 hours should be instituted the day following surgery. A solution consisting of one level teaspoon of table salt in an 8 oz. glass of warm water is recommended; however, you may select any of the commercial mouthwashes. Continue the rinses, at least following meals, until the sutures are removed.

5. Eat soft foods only for the first 24 hours and avoid chewing in the operated area until the sutures are removed. Do not stretch your lip unnecessarily or undergo excessive facial muscle movements.

6. Brush all of your teeth after each meal, taking care to avoid the sutured area. Food trapped around the sutures should be removed with a damp cotton swab. Proper cleansing prevents infection and the objectionable odors and taste that commonly follow surgical procedures.

7. Proper nourishment is necessary for optimum healing. Since many normal foods are difficult to chew, a diet of eggs, salads, and soups should be supplemented with high protein instant breakfast drinks and multivitamins. Avoid smoking and the use of alcoholic beverages.

8. If prescribed, take pain medication and antibiotics as instructed. It is important to return for the removal of your sutures as appointed. Be sure to call our office if you have any questions or if any irregularities occur.

(From Ingle JI and Taintor JF. *Endodontics*, 3rd ed. Philadelphia, Lee & Febiger, 1985.)

Suture Removal

Non-absorbable sutures should be removed after 5-7 days. To prevent discomfort place topical anesthetic along the incision line prior to removing the sutures. Use a sharp, pointed pair of scissors and carefully slide the scissor point under the suture. An alternative method is to slide an explorer tip under the suture and cut it with a #15 blade or to use a #11 or #12 blade to cut the suture.

Healing of the periapical area is evaluated radiograpically after six months and thereafter on a regular basis. By six months, bone should have regenerated in the apical area. Rowe[36] has shown that inflammatory cells can still be present in the apical region despite radiologic evidence of healing. However, as long as the patient has a firm, symptom-free, functional tooth with satisfactory 6-18 month postoperative radiographs, there is clinical success.

Factors That Minimize Surgical Morbidity

1. Avoid excessive trauma during the procedure since it contributes to increased pain, trismus, edema, possible infection, bone necrosis and sloughing, ecchymosis, and other complications.
2. Keep surgical time to a minimum.
3. Be very careful during reflection (active) and retraction (passive).
4. Use saline irrigation to lessen heat buildup and to cleanse the area.

   Heat produced during bone removal is a function of bur design, bur speed, pressure, and irrigation. Irrigation maintains temperatures in a safe range and prevents necrosis and sloughing.[3]

Some patient management ideas

- nitrous oxide
- audio analgesia
- sleeping medication the night before
- preoperative oral sedative medication
- IV sedation
- long-acting local anesthetic
- xylocaine into involved tissue around the apex to help eliminate pain during the procedure[3]
- nonsteroidal anti-inflammatory (NSAI) agents or moderate narcotic analgesics such as hydrocodone with acetaminophen

Table 4-9. Treatment plan.

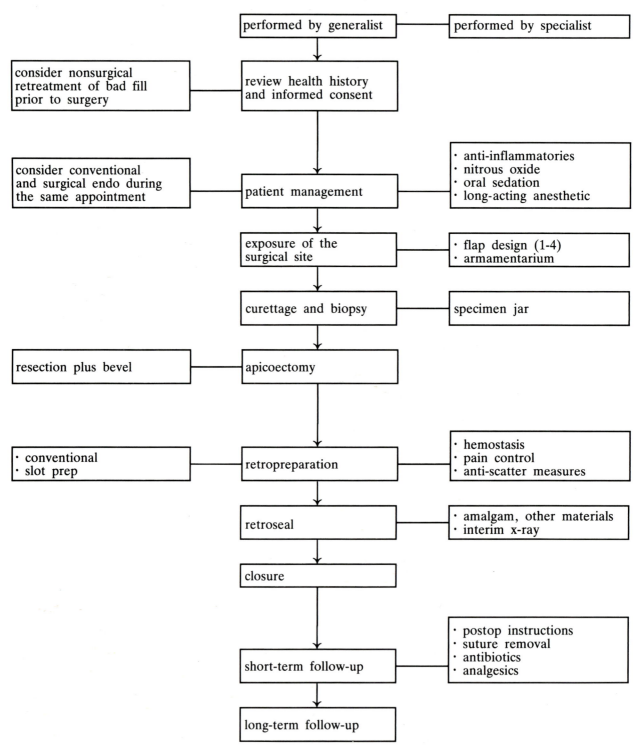

APICOECTOMY AND RETROSEAL FLOWCHART

| | performed by generalist | performed by specialist |

consider nonsurgical retreatment of bad fill prior to surgery — review health history and informed consent

consider conventional and surgical endo during the same appointment — patient management — · anti-inflammatories · nitrous oxide · oral sedation · long-acting anesthetic

exposure of the surgical site — · flap design (1-4) · armamentarium

curettage and biopsy — specimen jar

resection plus bevel — apicoectomy

· conventional · slot prep — retropreparation — · hemostasis · pain control · anti-scatter measures

retroseal — · amalgam, other materials · interim x-ray

closure

short-term follow-up — · postop instructions · suture removal · antibiotics · analgesics

long-term follow-up

CLINICAL CASES
Case 1
Maxillary Incisor Apicoectomy: Symptomatic but Without Periapical Lesion

Fig. 4-11, a. This 21-year-old female college student presented with nagging symptoms from tooth #8. The root canal and the crown had been done about one year before. Radiographically, there were no obvious signs of failure yet the tooth had continued to be sensitive to pressure and even ached frequently. The operator suggested nonsurgical endodontic retreatment to the patient. She was informed that it would require access through the existing crown and might weaken the crown. The dentist also told the patient that if the crown were to come off, subsequent treatment would include a post (which should have been done before the present crown was made), and a new crown. The patient did not like the proposed treatment plan and asked for alternatives. She accepted the periapical surgery option.

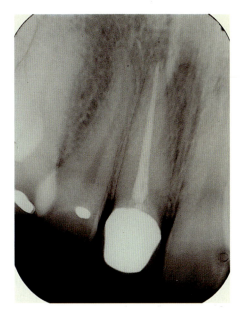

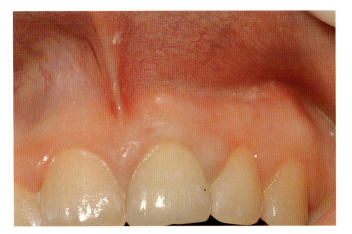

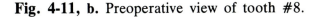

Fig. 4-11, b. Preoperative view of tooth #8.

Fig. 4-11, c. The operator selected a semilunar flap design to preserve marginal integrity and esthetics. Other factors contributed to this decision—normal periodontium, lack of root prominence, no suspected root exposure under soft tissue, and little or no bony defect. The apogee of the curve was made about 5 mm from the free margin. The median aspect of the incision was tucked underneath the frenum rather than going straight through it.

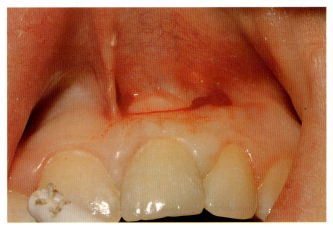

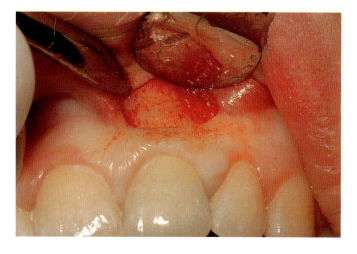

Fig. 4-11, d. Flap reflected. A full-thickness mucoperiosteal flap has been lifted, exposing bone. Access is conservative.

Fig. 4-11, e. Tooth-length was measured on the radiograph and this distance was then measured in the mouth with a sterile endodontic ruler. Bone was carefully removed in the area of the root apex and the yellowish dentinal color recognized. Sometimes it is quite difficult to distinguish tooth from bone. To verify the existence of root within the surgical field, the operator used his thumb and index finger to move the crown of the tooth back and forth. This created mobility at the apex that confirmed the location of the root apex. More root was removed until the gutta-percha was identified, thus confirming existing anatomy. Using the best possible clinical judgement, about 2 mm of the root apex were resected and then the root end was beveled about 45 degrees from the facial. All of this was accomplished with a straight handpiece and 702 bur. Note the adequate width of bone between the beveled portion of root and the incision line. The flap proved to be satisfactory in this case.

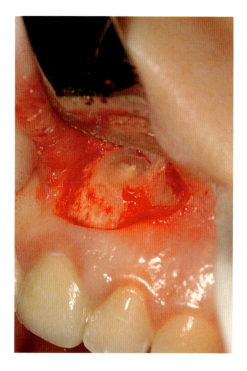

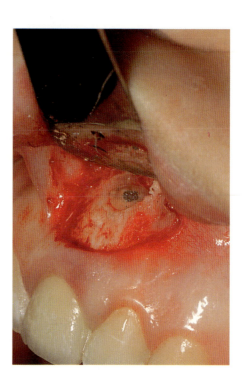

Fig. 4-11, f. A retropreparation was made extending about 2 mm into the end of the root in its long axis. A conventional dental contra-angle on a slow-speed straight handpiece was used with a #2 round bur. A zinc-free amalgam was used to seal.

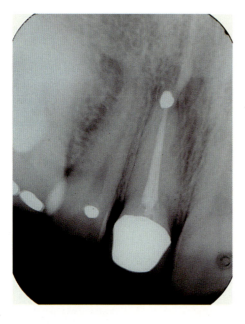

Fig. 4-11, g. Postoperative radiograph. Within one week the patient's symptoms subsided. She has remained pain-free for seven years.

Fig. 4-11, h. Black silk sutures (4.0 with fs-2 needle) were placed. The narrow isthmus area of gingiva labial to the crown was avoided to preserve vascularity and esthetics. Pressure was placed on the flap for about one minute to initiate fibrin adhesion. Suture removal was scheduled for five days postoperatively.

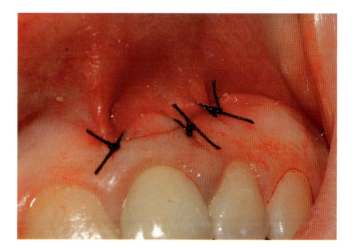

Case 2
Maxillary Canine Apicoectomy

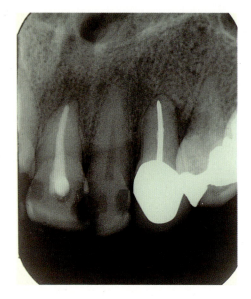

Fig. 4-12, a. This 45-year-old woman is a self-employed artist. The silver point fill on tooth #6 was performed 15 years before. It has recently become symptomatic. She was told that the treatment of choice was retrieval of the silver point through the lingual of the crown and nonsurgical retreatment with gutta-percha. The high probability that the crown would need to be redone was mentioned—if not soon, then within the next few years. She chose the surgical treatment option.

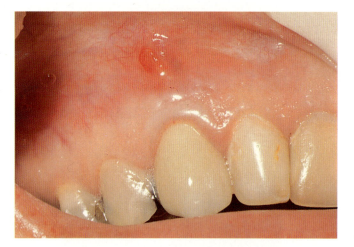

Fig. 4-12, b. Preoperative view showing fistulous tract near the apical region of the tooth.

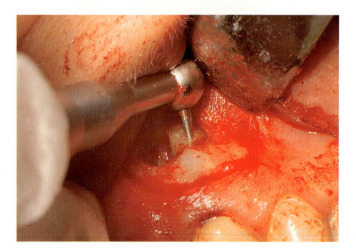

Fig. 4-12, c. A semilunar flap design was selected since there were no contraindications and it avoided manipulation of free marginal tissues covering the apical edge of the crown. After root-end resection, beveling, and removal of diseased tissue from the bony defect, a microhead handpiece and round bur were used to create a retropreparation.

Fig. 4-12, d. The amalgam retroseal has been accomplished. Note where the infection has eroded bone: more on the distal aspect of the root rather than at the apex. One week later, the tooth was extracted because of severe pain. A lateral canal, located at mid-root on the distal surface, was sealed and the tooth reimplanted. Since that time it has a 4-year history without problems.

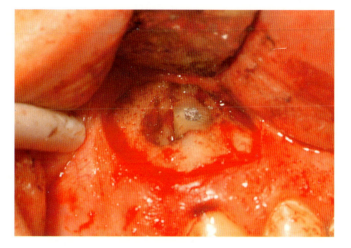

Fig. 4-12, e. Sutured flap. There is inflammation in the isthmus area of marginal gingiva and even slight cyanosis along the free margin. This was a concern until the five-day postop visit. This is one of the potential hazards with a semilunar flap design. If the apogee of the curved incision had been perhaps one millimeter further from the free margin, it would have been better. There are tradeoffs with each flap method that need to be weighed in each case.

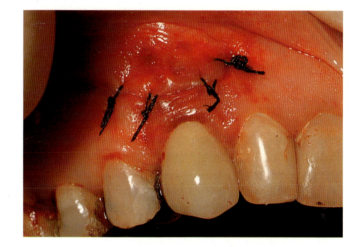

Fig. 4-12, f. Postoperative radiograph.

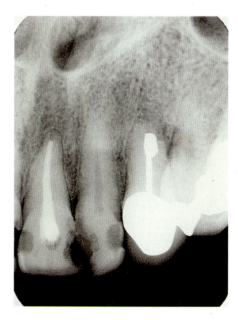

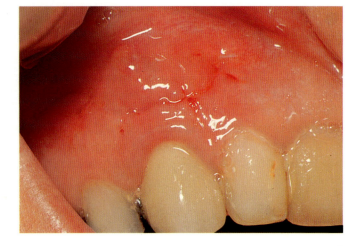

Fig. 4-12, g. Five-day postoperative view.

Case 3
Maxillary Incisor Apicoectomy: Endodontics and Apicoectomy Performed at Same Appointment

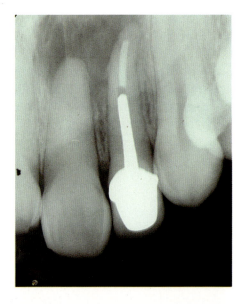

Fig. 4-13, a. Tooth #9 on this patient has a necrotic pulp which is responsible for a large, longstanding infection (about one centimeter in diameter). Only lately has the tooth become painful. The lesion is slow to respond to antibiotics. It has been opened to drain. The patient is under pressure at work: he cannot afford down-time from a tooth. It was decided to perform conventional endodontics *and* surgical endodontics (including removal of the infection) at the same appointment. If the procedure is done on Friday afternoon, he should be feeling well enough by Monday to return to work.

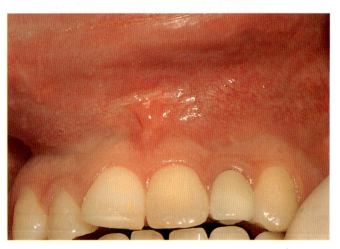

Fig. 4-13, b. Preoperative view. Before starting the surgery, endodontic access was created and the canal thoroughly instrumented. Seepage from infection prevented the operator from obtaining a dry canal.

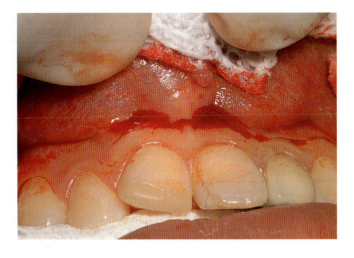

Fig. 4-13, c. In this case, the flap was a modified semilunar without the releasing components. Made entirely in attached gingiva, it is commonly referred to as an "attached gingiva" flap.

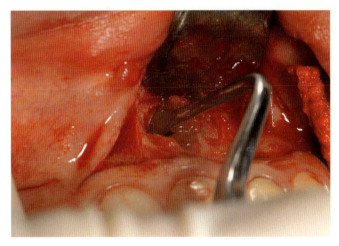

Fig. 4-13, d. A Seldin #23 retractor is holding the mucoperiosteal flap above the level of the bony defect. The incision was made laterally enough to allow tissue flexibility that affords adequate access. A surgical spoon curette is being used to remove granulomatous tissue from around the root apex.

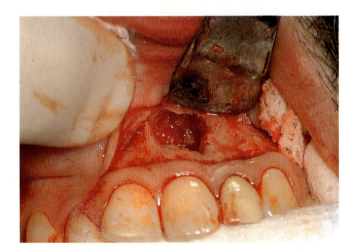

Fig. 4-13, e. The defect has been debrided and the root apex, protruding upward into the hollowness, has been resected. The bevel has also been made.

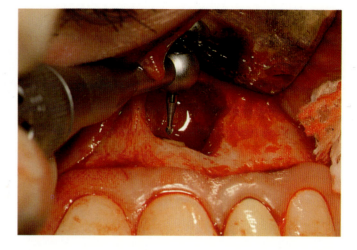

Fig. 4-13, f. The microhead handpiece with a round bur is being positioned for making the retropreparation.

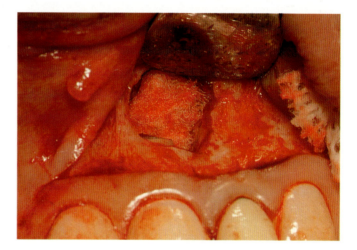

Fig. 4-13, g. Cotton has been packed into the defect to help with hemostasis, and to act as a filter to catch any loose amalgam scraps. Cotton is being phased out of use by most practitioners because of complications in healing with residual fibers left behind in the surgical site.

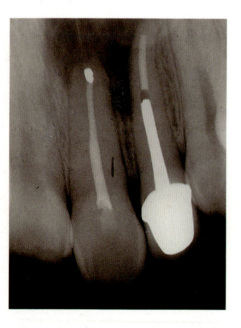

Fig. 4-13, h. Postoperative radiograph. The entire procedure took approximately 40 minutes.

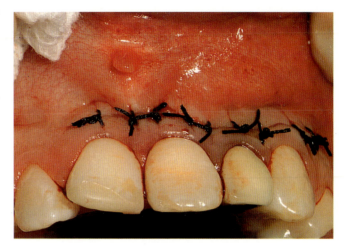

Fig. 4-13, i. Sutured flap.

Case 4
Maxillary Incisor Apicoectomy:
Apicoectomy and Periodontal Surgery
Performed at Same Time

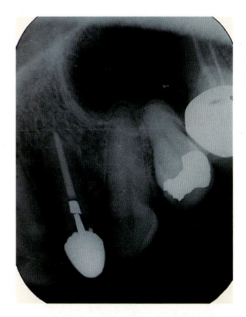

Fig. 4-14, a. The preoperative radiograph of tooth #7 reveals metal in the canal apical to a short post. The metal object and post effectively block canal access from a coronal approach.

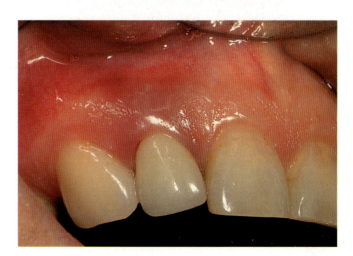

Fig. 4-14, b. In addition to needing endodontic surgery, there is also a localized periodontal problem on the labial of the tooth. Gingival tissues are swollen and cyanotic. Probing produced a reading of 5 mm. Because of the periodontal situation, it was decided to use a triangular flap design.

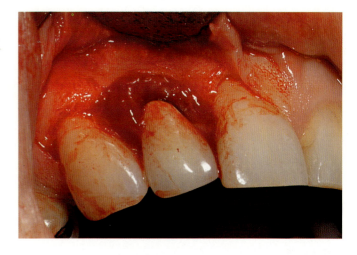

Fig. 4-14, c. Note the granulomatous tissue along the labial root surface of the tooth.

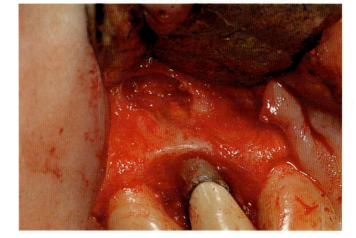

Fig. 4-14, d. Pathologic tissue was removed with a periodontal curette, exposing the periapical defect. A bony ledge was created by infection on the labial of teeth #'s 6 and 7.

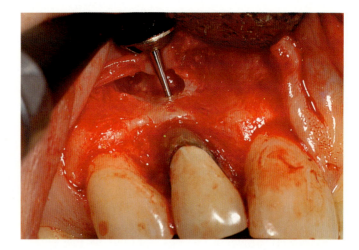

Fig. 4-14, e. Resection of the apex and beveling have been done. The retropreparation is being made with a microhead handpiece. A #6 round bur was used to smooth out the bony ledge mentioned in **d.**

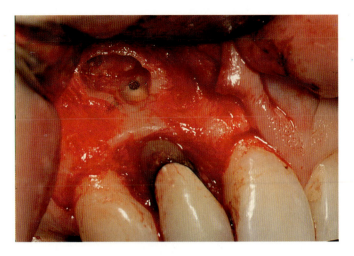

Fig. 4-14, f. A retroamalgam has been placed.

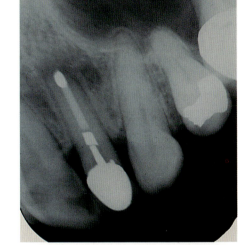

Fig. 4-14, g. Postoperative radiograph.

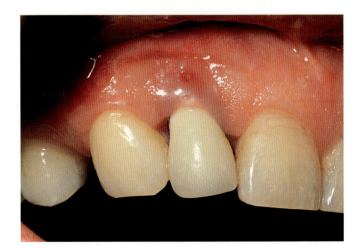

Fig. 4-14, h. The six months postoperative radiograph shows bone loss on the facial surface of the tooth. A root fracture was diagnosed. It will eventually need to be extracted.

Case 5
Maxillary Incisor Apicoectomy:
Longstanding Fibrotic Lesion

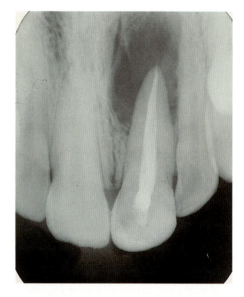

Fig. 4-15, a. Preoperative radiograph. This 19-year-old man is leaving the country in about one month. Endodontics was recently completed on tooth #8, but symptoms have not subsided. To eliminate the chance of future flare-up, endodontic surgery was chosen. This is obviously a lesion of longstanding duration.

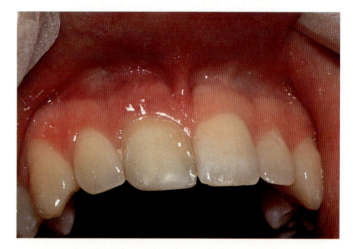

Fig. 4-15, b. Preoperative view.

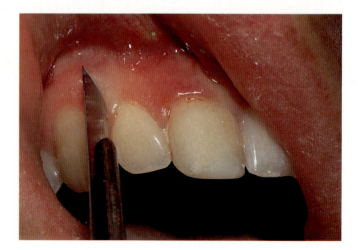

Fig. 4-15, c. Because of the size of the lesion, a semilunar flap is contraindicated. If used, the incision would have been directly over the defect and not supported with solid bone.

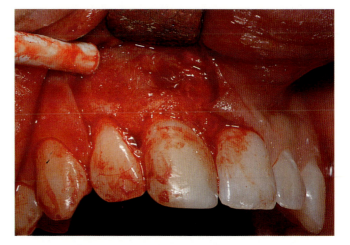

Fig. 4-15, d. Flap in the process of being reflected.

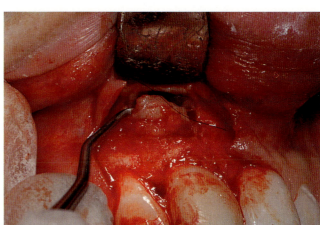

Fig. 4-15, e. Bone did not have to be removed with a bur since it had already been destroyed by the infection. The periapical tissue is dense and fibrotic. A periodontal curette is being used to remove diseased tissue.

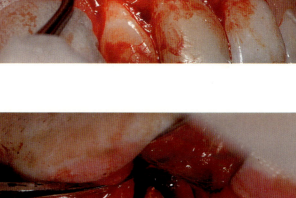

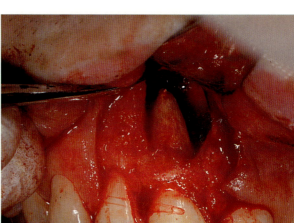

Fig. 4-15, f. Some of the periapical soft tissue is removed in order to visualize the root. Here we clearly see the root tip extending into the hollowness of the bony defect.

Fig. 4-15, g. Once access is improved by resecting the root tip and then beveling it, the remainder of the diseased tissue can be eliminated.

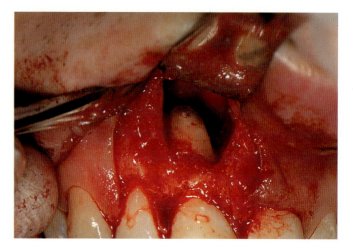

Fig. 4-15, h. Gauze strips were placed in the defect to promote hemostasis and to prevent amalgam from getting lost in the defect.

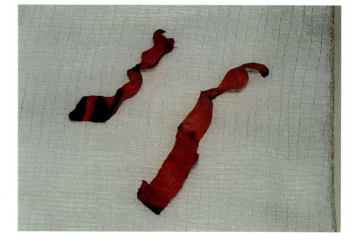

Fig. 4-15, i. Sutured case.

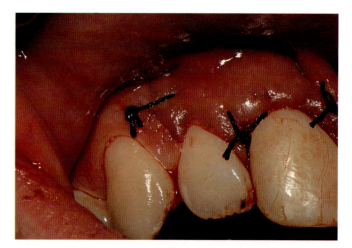

Fig. 4-15, j. Postoperative radiograph. Even though the retrofill is clinically acceptable, it is not ideal in that it was not made completely in the long axis of the tooth.

Case 6
Maxillary Premolar Apicoectomy

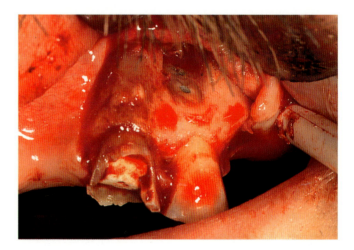

Fig. 4-16. Maxillary first premolar. The retroamalgams have been placed (buccal and lingual) and the case is ready for closure.

Case 7
Maxillary First Molar Apicoectomy

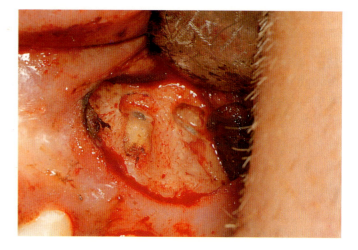

Fig. 4-17, a. A semilunar flap design allows access to the buccal roots of this maxillary first molar. The case is ready for closure. Part of the mesiobuccal root protruded through cortical bone. It has been shaved back to be contained with normal bone contours.

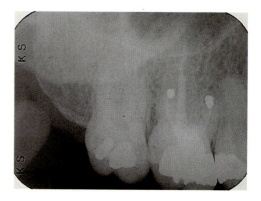

Fig. 4-17, b. Postoperative radiograph.

Case 8
Maxillary First Molar Apicoectomy

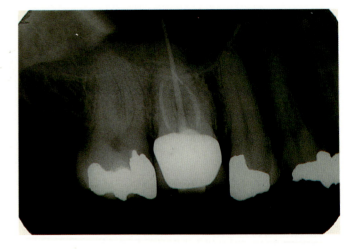

Fig. 4-18, a. Preoperative radiograph of tooth #14.

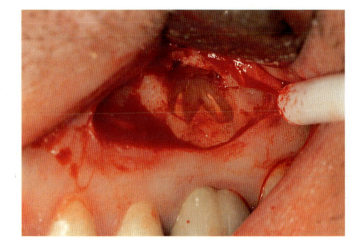

Fig. 4-18, b. A semilunar flap gives adequate access to buccal roots. After resection and beveling, the gutta-percha fills are visible.

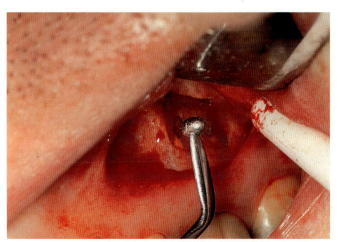

Fig. 4-18, c. With retropreparations completed, amalgam is being transported to the surgical site. Some operators prefer using a tiny ball of fresh amalgam on the end of a small carving instrument instead of an amalgam carrier.

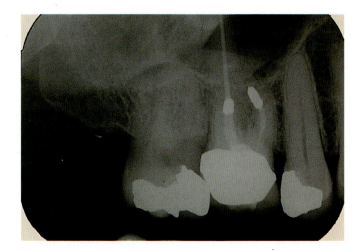

Fig. 4-18, d. Postoperative radiograph of the completed case.

References

1. Arens DE, Adams WR, DeCastro RA. *Endodontic Surgery*. Philadelphia, Pa: Harper & Row; 1981.

2. Burke IT. Retro root filling. *Oral Surg Oral Med Oral Pathol*. 1979;48:254.

3. Ingle JI, Taintor JF. *Endodontics*. 3rd ed. Philadelphia, Pa: Lee & Febiger; 1985.

4. Lewis RD, Block RM. Management of endodontic failures. *Oral Surg Oral Med Oral Pathol*. 1988;66(6):711.

5. Schoeffel GJ. The apicoectomy myth: failures need surgery. *Dent Today*. 1989; March:40-41.

6. Skoglund A, Persson G. A follow-up study of apicoectomized teeth with total loss of the buccal bone plate. *Oral Surg Oral Med Oral Pathol*. 1985;59:78.

7. Green D. Stereomicroscopic study of the root apices of 400 maxillary and mandibular teeth. *Oral Surg Oral Med Oral Pathol*. 1956;9:1224.

8. Neaverth EJ, Kotley LM, Kaltenbach RF. Clinical Investigation (in vivo) of endodontically treated maxillary first molars. *J Endodontics*. 1987;13(10):505.

9. Kruger GO. *Oral and Maxillofacial Surgery*. 6th ed. St Louis, Mo: The CV Mosby Co; 1984.

10. Morse DR, Bhambhani SM. A dentist's dilemma: Nonsurgical endodontic therapy or periapical surgery for teeth with apparent pulpal pathosis and an associated periapical radiolucent lesion. *Oral Surg Oral Med Oral Pathol*. 1990;70(3):333.

11. Miserendino LJ. The laser apicoectomy: Endodontic application of the CO_2 laser for periapical surgery. *Oral Surg Oral Med Oral Pathol*. 1988;66(5):615.

12. Abdal AK, Retief DH. The apical seal via the retrosurgical approach. *Oral Surg Oral Med Oral Pathol*. 1982;53:614.

13. Harrison JW, Todd MJ. The effect of root resection on the sealing property of root canal obturations. *Oral Surg Oral Med Oral Pathol*. 1980;50:264.

14. Saad AY, Clem WH. The use of radiographs in periapical surgery. *Oral Surg Oral Med Oral Pathol*. 1990;69(3):361.

15. Barry GN, Heyman RA, Elias A. Comparison of apical sealing methods. *Oral Surg Oral Med Oral Pathol*. 1975;39:806.

16. Nelson LW, Mahler DB. Factors influencing the sealing behavior of retrograde amalgam fillings. *Oral Surg Oral Med Oral Pathol*. 1990;69(3):356.

17. Tronstad L, et al. Sealing ability of dental amalgams as retrograde fillings in endodontic therapy. *J Endo*. 1983;9:551.

18. Birn H, Winther JE. *Manual of Minor Oral Surgery. A Step-by-Step Atlas*. Philadelphia, Pa: The WB Saunders Co; 1982.

19. Laskin DM. *Oral and Maxillofacial Surgery*, Vol. 2. St Louis, Mo: The CV Mosby Co; 1985.

20. Grossman LI. *Endodontic Practice*, 10th ed. Philadelphia, Pa: Lea & Febiger; 1981:348-383.

21. Bramwell JD. Sealing ability of four retrofilling techniques. *J Endo*. 1986;12:95.

22. Barry GN, et al. Sealing quality of polycarboxylate cements when compared to amalgam as retrofilling material. *Oral Surg Oral Med Oral Pathol*. 1976;42:109.

23. Negm MM. The effect of varnish and pit and fissure sealants on the sealing capacity of retrofilling techniques. *Oral Surg Oral Med Oral Pathol*. 1988;66(4):483.

24. Alexander SA. Spontaneous expulsion of a retrograde filling. *Oral Surg Oral Med Oral Pathol*. 1983;56:321.

25. Bondra DL, et al. Leakage in vitro with IRM, high copper amalgam, and EBA cement as retrofilling materials. *J Endo*. 1989;15(4):157.

26. Dorn SO, Gartner AH. Retrograde filling materials: a retrospective success-failure study of amalgam, EMA, IRM. *J Endo*. 1990;16(8):391.

27. Barkhordar RA, Pelzner RB, Stark MM. Use of glass ionomers as retrofilling materials. *Oral Surg*. 1989;67(6):734.

28. Zetterqvist L, Anneroth G, Nordenram A. Glass ionomer cement as retrograde filling material. *Int J Oral Maxillofac Surg*. 1987;16:459.

29. Thirawat J, Edmunds DH. The sealing ability of materials used as retrograde root fillings in endodontic surgery. *Int Endo J.* 1989;22:295.

30. Waikakul A. Punwutikorn J. Gold leaf as an alternative retrograde filling material. *Oral Surg Oral Med Oral Pathol.* 1989;67(6):746.

31. MacPherson MG, et al. Leakage in vitro with high-temperature thermoplasticized gutta-percha, high copper amalgam, and warm gutta-percha when used as retrofilling materials. *J Endo.* 1989;15(5):212.

32. Escobar C, et al. A comparative study between injectable low temperature (70 degree C.) gutta-percha and silver amalgam as a retroseal. *Oral Surg Oral Med Oral Pathol.* 1986;61(5):504.

33. Amagasa T, et al. Apicoectomy with retrograde gutta-percha root filling. *Oral Surg Oral Med Oral Pathol.* 1989;68(3):339.

34. High AS, Russell JL. Retrograde root filling using antibiotic-containing, radiopaque, bone cement. *J Dent.* 1988;17:241.

35. Tanzilli JP, et al. A comparison of the marginal adaptation of retrograde techniques: a scanning electron microscopic study. *Oral Surg Oral Med Oral Pathol.* 1980;50:74.

36. Rowe AHR. Post extraction histology of root resection. *Dent Pract.* 1967;17:343.

Additional Reading Material

1. Finne K, et al. Retrograde root filling with amalgam and Cavit. *Oral Surg Oral Med Oral Pathol.* 1977;43:621.

2. Gerstein H. Inter-relationship between endodontic treatment and periodontic and restorative treatment. In Goldman HM, et al, editors: *Current Therapy in Dentistry.* Vol 5. St Louis, Mo: The CV Mosby Co; 1974.

3. Luks S. Root and amalgam techniques in the practice of endodontics. *JADA.* 1956;53:424.

4. Stabholz A, et al. Marginal adaptation of retrograde fillings and its correlation with sealability. *J Endo.* 1985;11:218.

5. Weine FS. *Endodontic Therapy.* 3rd ed. St Louis, Mo: The CV Mosby Co; 1982.

Chapter 5

Intentional Replantation

INTRODUCTION

Intentional replantation is generally considered a procedure of last resort to save a functionally sound tooth that would otherwise be lost. It is indicated when conventional endodontic therapy has failed, when it is impossible to perform conventional endodontic treatment, or when endodontic surgery is not practical.[1,2,3] Tables 5-1 and 5-2 elaborate more fully on indications and contraindications. In essence, intentional replantation involves a tooth being purposefully removed from the mouth, careful manipulation of tooth and socket, and then replantation in the socket. Success rates vary among clinicians, but the general consensus is that the less time the tooth is out of the mouth the greater the postoperative longevity. Most recommend no longer than 10-15 minutes, with 30 minutes being the limit at which one would still predict a successful outcome over an extended period of time.

Diagnostic Criteria

Table 5-1. Indications for Intentional Replantation

Intentional replantations are generally performed with posterior teeth on which apicoectomies and retroseals cannot be done, and which would need to be extracted anyway.

  1. Replantations are generally performed on symptomatic teeth with:
- calcified canals
- curved or dilacerated canals that cannot be instrumented
- a broken instrument lodged in the canal or projecting beyond the root apex
- an inaccessible perforation
- a nonremovable silver point
- apices near nerves that could be damaged from periapical surgery

  2. The teeth should have a normal periodontium.

  3. The patient should understand the procedure and be in favor of it.

Table 5-2. Contraindications for Intentional Replantation

1. Unhealthy periodontium
2. Inappropriate root conditions
   - divergent roots
   - dilacerated roots
   - hypercementosis
   - suspected ankylosis
3. Nonrestorable tooth
4. Weak tooth (such a tooth can be provisionally strengthened prior to surgery)
5. Poor oral hygiene
6. Lack of acceptance by the patient

Even though there may initially be a good prognosis for the procedure, the situation can deteriorate because of adverse conditions during surgery. Examples of these situations are listed in Table 5-3.

Table 5-3. Potential Surgical Problems that can Compromise Success

1. Tooth out of the mouth too long[1]
   Optimum: 10-15 minutes
   - under 30 minutes - about 10% root resorption
   - over 2 hours - 95% root resorption
2. Root fracture
3. Crown fracture
4. Bone fracture
5. Bone expansion and subsequent rapid relapse to its original position, preventing replantation
6. Bone burnishing from excessive tooth manipulation during surgery
7. Drying of the tooth
8. Abrasion of the coronal part of the root with a forcep
9. Failure to remove periapical pathology
10. Removal of the residual periodontal ligament lining the socket or the tooth

SURGICAL TREATMENT

Operative Technique

Preoperative Preparations:

1. It is better if conventional endodontic treatment has already been completed. Note: This can also be done intraoperatively, while the tooth is out of the mouth, or a month or so postoperatively.

2. Patients requiring scaling should have it completed several days before the procedure.

3. The patient should already have been apprised of advantages and disadvantages of the procedure (informed consent received).

4. All anticipated armamentaria should be assembled.

Operative Procedures:

1. Carefully reflect cervical gingiva.

2. Use an elevator to gently luxate the tooth.

3. Further luxate and then extract with forcep.

4. Temporarily place the tooth in a receptacle containing sterile saline, or better yet, Hank's solution (similar to isotonic media used for organ transplants).

5. Carefully curette away pathological tissue at the base of the socket.

6. Hold the tooth, using gauze impregnated with an isotonic solution.

7. If endodontic therapy has not been completed, do so at this time or schedule for a later date. Teeth that are not treated endodontically are more susceptible to root resorption.

8. Resect 2-3 mm off the end of the root (see Fig. 5-1). This helps eliminate possible lateral canals, avoids the problem of foramina not at the apex, rids the tooth of apical curves, and gives better visualization of the canals.

9. Bevel the sharp edge formed by the apical resection. This reduces trauma to socket walls on reinsertion (Fig. 5-2).

10. Create an apical retropreparation into the canal (in the long axis of the tooth) about 2-3 mm deep and 1 mm in diameter (Fig. 5-2).

11. Fill the retropreparation with zinc-free amalgam or another acceptable retrosealing material and rinse the tooth.

12. Suction the clot from the socket.

13. Finger pressure should be applied facially and lingually to reapproximate bone that may have been expanded during the extraction process. **Replant the tooth back in its socket within 10-15 minutes.** If the tooth is still out of the socket after 30 minutes, thought should be given to aborting the replantation procedure because of ligament desiccation and anticipated root resorption.

14. Relieve the occlusion so that the tooth is slightly out of contact.

15. Splint the tooth to adjacent teeth if it exhibits sufficient mobility (see Figs. 5-3 and 5-4). Remove the splint in two weeks.

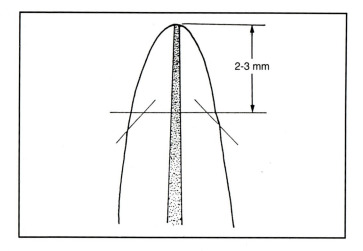

Fig. 5-1. Resection of the root apex prior to replantation.

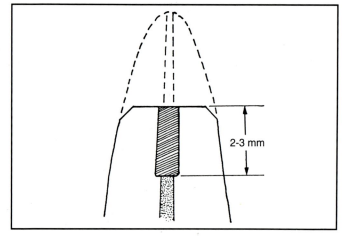

Fig. 5-2. Retroseal performed prior to replantation.

Splinting of Replanted Teeth

Some mobility is a natural consequence of the procedure, but especially with molars, it is not usually sufficient to warrant splinting. If, however, the operator feels excessive mobility may jeopardize the prognosis, then splinting should be done. Figures 5-3 and 5-4 illustrate one splinting method.

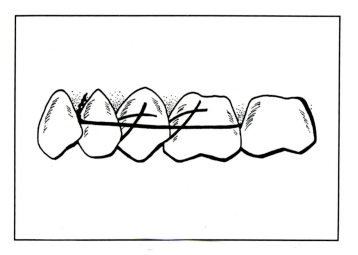

Fig. 5-3. A single piece of wire, such as .014 orthodontic ligature wire, is placed facially and lingually to the replanted tooth and one tooth on either side (mesially and distally). Ends are joined, twisted, and tucked into a facial embrasure.

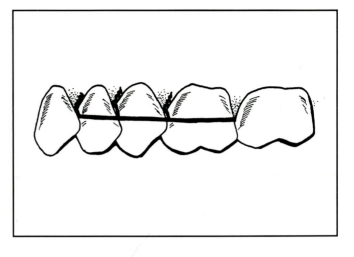

Fig. 5-4. Two shorter pieces are positioned above and below the contacts mesial and distal to the replanted tooth, and then they are twisted and tucked into adjacent embrasures.

Postoperative Care

1. Administer antibiotics and analgesics.
2. Give postoperative instructions, including the following:
   - Do not chew on the tooth for one week.
   - Do not brush the tooth for a few days. Instead, clean with a washcloth.
   - On the day after surgery, rinse with warm saline 3-4 times a day (1 tsp. salt in a glass of water).
   - Take medications as directed.
3. Examine the patient after one week to evaluate healing and then again after two weeks.
4. Take an x-ray and gently probe sulcus depths at six weeks.
5. X-ray and evaluate every six months for two years.

Healing is generally uneventful. Pain is moderate and subsides within a few days to one week. There is slight mobility for about two to three weeks. After one month, most teeth have regained their original stability.

Discussion

Grossman[2] has reported successful cases that he has followed for up to 20 years. Koenig[1] reported an 82% success rate with 192 cases which were followed for 4.5 years. Most of the failures occurred within the first year. This finding was a confirmation of work previously done in the 60s[4], and 70s[5]. When failed teeth were extracted and examined in Koenig's study, none of them showed signs of clinical ankylosis. Primary causes of failure were:

• breakdown of periapical or periodontal bone (or both)	62.5%
• external root resorption	25%
• severe discomfort or tooth fracture	12.5%

Intentional replantation is not commonly performed, yet there is a place for it in modern dentistry. The case prognosis improves with prudent patient selection and adherence to sound surgical techniques, including time restraints. Both radiographic and clinical studies confirm that successfully reimplanted teeth are firm in the socket, show little or no root or bone resorption, have normal sulcus depths, and have normal looking gingiva. These teeth are asymptomatic and functional. The procedure should be a part of the dentist's surgical repertoire.

Table 5-4. Intentional Replantation Flow Chart

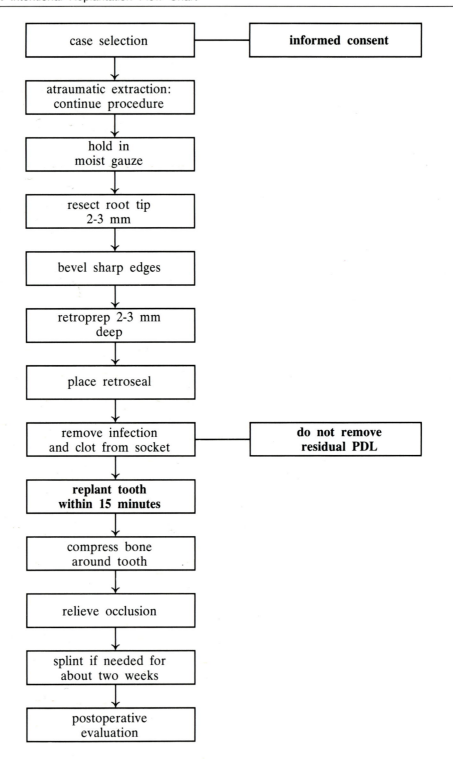

CLINICAL CASES
Case 1
Postendodontic Replantation

Fig. 5-5, a. This is the radiograph of a 55-year-old woman who had had endodontic therapy completed on tooth #4 about two years before. It has remained symptomatic ever since. She insisted on extraction.

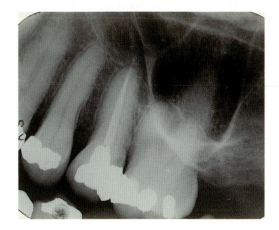

Fig. 5-5, b. Preoperative clinical view.

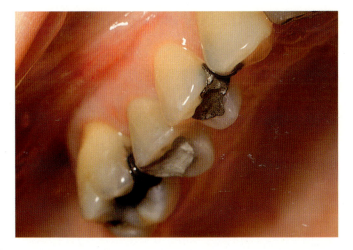

Fig. 5-5, c. The tooth was luxated and is now being carefully extracted.

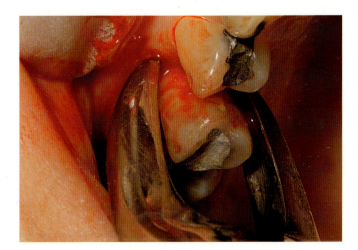

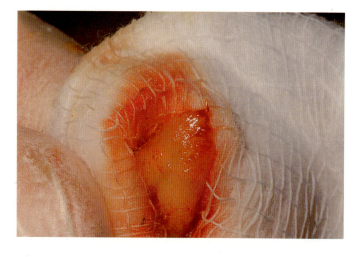

Fig. 5-5, d. The tooth is examined briefly prior to manipulation and replantation.

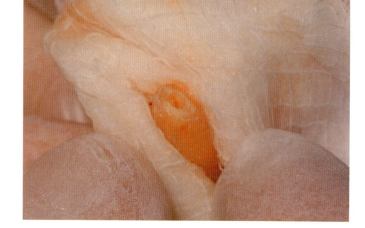

Fig. 5-5, e. Resection and retropreparation completed.

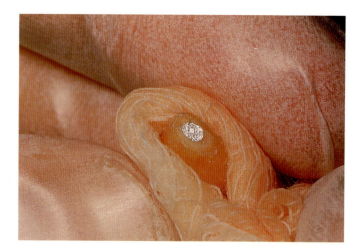

Fig. 5-5, f. Retroseal performed with zinc-free amalgam.

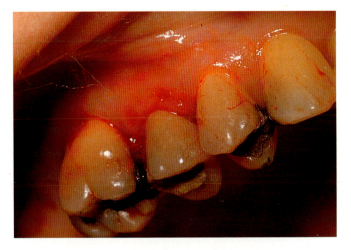

Fig. 5-5, g. Replantation.

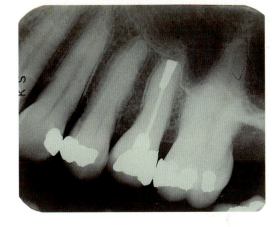

Fig. 5-5, h. Postoperative x-ray. This tooth is still asymptomatic and in function after four years.

Case 2
Extraction, Endodontics Outside the Mouth, and Replantation

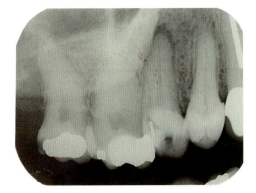

Fig. 5-6, a. Because of extreme pain, this patient, a 45-year-old woman, has requested that #13 be extracted. This is the preoperative x-ray.

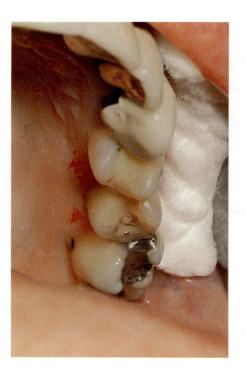

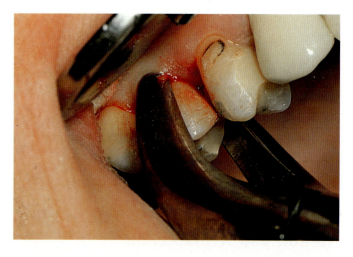

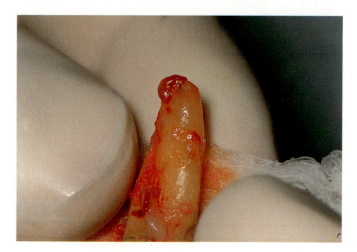

Fig. 5-6, b. Preoperative clinical view.

Fig. 5-6, c. Extraction.

Fig. 5-6, d. Extracted tooth. Because of the ease of removal, the option of intentional replantation was presented to the patient.

Fig. 5-6, e. The tooth was quickly instrumented, dried, and filled by pulling gutta-percha through the apex.

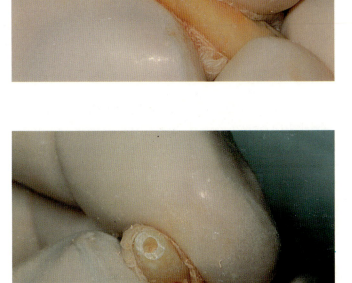

Fig. 5-6, f. Resection and retropreparation.

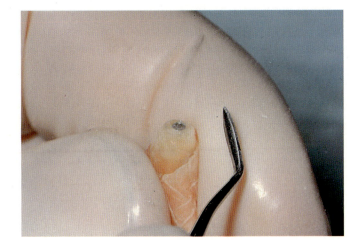

Fig. 5-6, g. Retroseal.

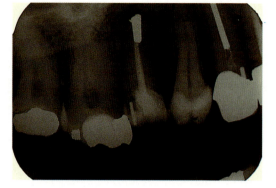

Fig. 5-6, h. Postoperative x-ray. After three years this tooth is still asymptomatic and in function.

Case 3
Extraction, Sealing of a Canal Without Endodontics, and Replantation

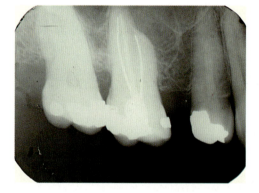

Fig. 5-7, a. When this 52-year-old woman presented with the complaint of pain from tooth #14, it was explained that endodontic retreatment was indicated. She refused and demanded that the tooth be extracted.

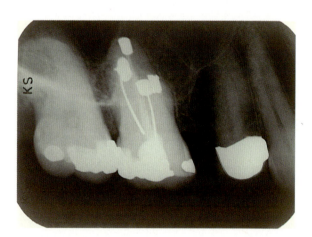

Fig. 5-7, b. Once the tooth was out, she was given the chance for it to be replanted. A second mesiobuccal root was observed and all four roots were sealed. This approach was somewhat risky in that the fourth root contained necrotic material that was not extirpated and could jeopardize the prognosis. This x-ray gives a five-year postoperative view of a tooth that has remained asymptomatic.

Case 4
Fourteen and Eight Year
Postoperative Radiographs

Fig. 5-8, a. This is the x-ray from an 87-year-old woman who was 75 years old when she first presented with a periapical abscess associated with tooth #18. Originally, there was a purulent exudate draining from the distal of #18 into the mouth and the tooth was extremely painful. It was extracted, the tooth was prepared, and a retroseal was placed. A crown was placed six months later. This is a 14-year follow-up x-ray. Some external root resorption is evident on the distal, but it has remained unchanged since the first year.

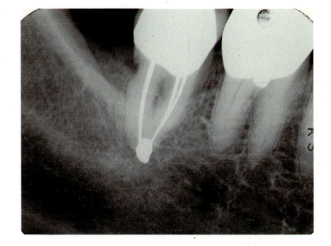

Fig. 5-8, b. Tooth #15 has been successfully replanted. It was extracted and replaced in the socket eight years prior to this x-ray being taken. Conical roots lend themselves most favorably to the procedure.

Case 5
Contraindication for Replantation

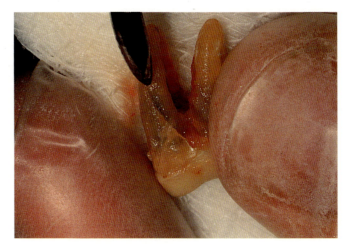

Fig. 5-9. Extracted tooth once considered for replantation. It was discarded due to the vertical fracture.

Case 6
Replantation of Mandibular Second Molar with Serious Infection

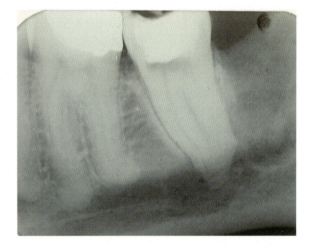

Fig. 5-10, a. Preoperative radiograph. The patient, a 35-year-old man, presented with a painful tooth (#31).

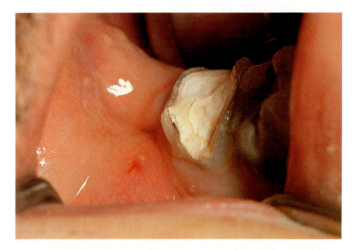

Fig. 5-10, b. Endodontic therapy had been initiated one year before, but was never completed. Periapical infection was exerting pressure on the inferior alveolar nerve, causing paresthesia of the right lower lip.

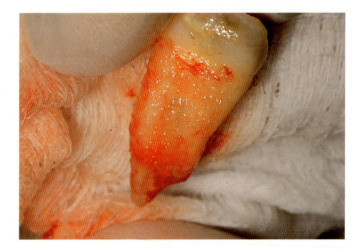

Fig. 5-10, c. After two weeks of antibiotics and unsuccessful endodontic therapy (the discomfort and nerve dysesthesia were now both worsening), the tooth was extracted.

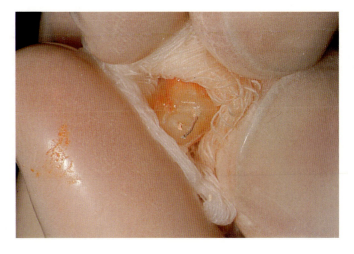

Fig. 5-10, d. Canals were debrided, dried, lined with sealer, and filled with gutta-percha.

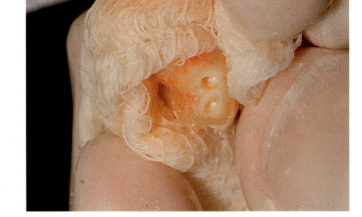

Fig. 5-10, e. Root resection and retropreparation.

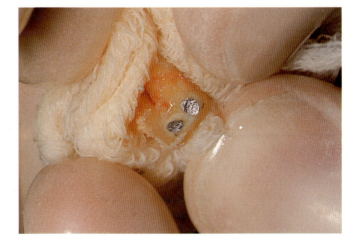

Fig. 5-10, f. Retroseal.

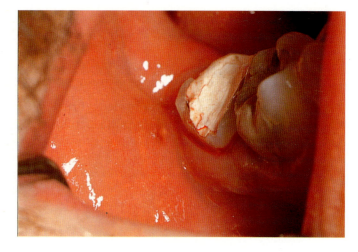

Fig. 5-10, g. Replantation.

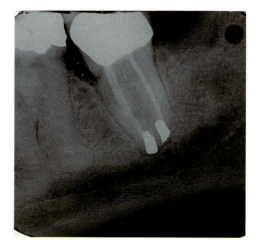

Fig. 5-10, h. Postoperative x-ray taken two years postoperatively. There is a five millimeter pocket on the mesial; however, the tooth is asymptomatic.

Case 7
Replantation of Maxillary Molar With Divergent Roots

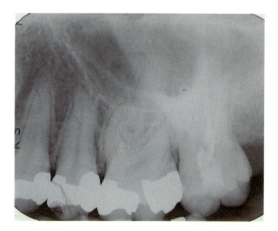

Fig. 5-11, a. This patient is experiencing severe pain from tooth #2 and does not want retreatment.

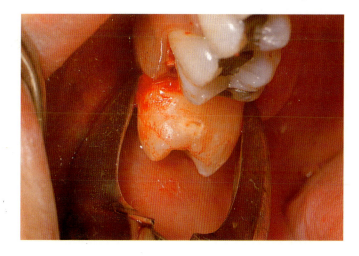

Fig. 5-11, b. Atraumatic extraction.

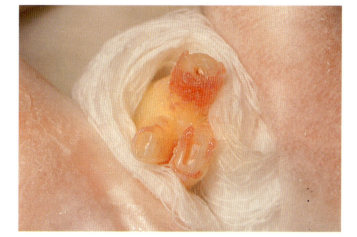

Fig. 5-11, c. Extracted tooth wrapped in saline-impregnated gauze.

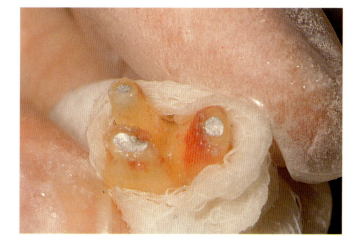

Fig. 5-11, d. Sealed roots.

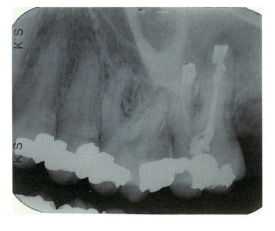

Fig. 5-11, e. X-ray of replanted tooth taken three years postoperatively. After three years, the tooth is still in the mouth and there are no signs of failure.

Case 8
Replantation Case with 14-Year Follow-up

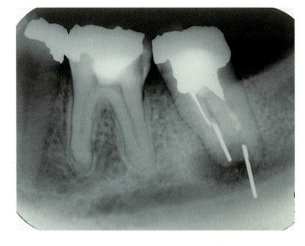

Fig. 5-12, a. In the process of placing a sectional silver point in the distal canal, the point was inadvertently overextended into periapical tissues.

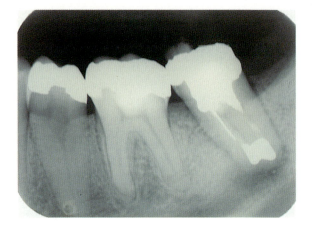

Fig. 5-12, b. Ten years later, a general dentist and an endodontist collaborated to perform the replantation procedure.

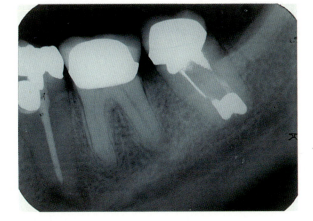

Fig. 5-12, c. Three-year postoperative check.

Fig. 5-12, d. Thirteen years postoperatively, the tooth has been crowned and periapical bone appears healthy. The tooth has been asymptomatic since shortly after it was replanted. X-rays are used with permission from Dr. John Young.

Case 9
Replantation Failure: Apical Resorption

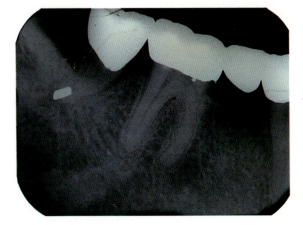

Fig. 5-13, a. Replanted tooth.

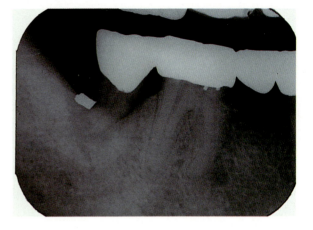

Fig. 5-13, b. After three years, the tooth is mobile and tender to chewing pressure. Obvious failure of the replantation procedure will require an extraction in the near future. This patient has habits of clenching and bruxing.

Case 10
Replantation Failure:
Lateral Resorption

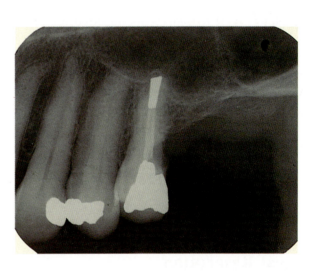

Fig. 5-14, a. The patient presented with pain emanating from this maxillary premolar that had been replanted three years previously.

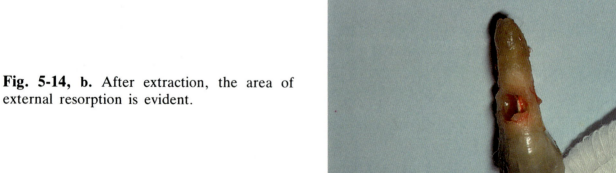

Fig. 5-14, b. After extraction, the area of external resorption is evident.

References

1. Koenig KH, Nguyen NT, Barkhorday RA. Intentional replantation: a report of 192 cases. *Gen Dent*. 1988;Jul/Aug:327.

2. Grossman LI. Intentional replantation of teeth: A clinical evaluation. *JADA*. 1982;104(5):633.

3. Din FM. Intentional replantation to prevent loss of an abutment tooth. *Gen Dent*. 1987;35(1):39.

4. Andraesen JO, Hjorting-Hansen E. Replantation of teeth. II. Histological study of 22 replanted anterior teeth in humans. *Acta Odont Scand*. 1966;24:287.

5. Hansen J, Fibaek B. Clinical experience of auto- and allotransplantation of teeth. *Int Dent J*. 1972;22:270.

Chapter 6

Orthodontic Brackets On Unerupted Teeth

INTRODUCTION

Permanent teeth that fail to erupt in a timely manner are a concern to dentists, patients, and parents. The most common tooth to be delayed in eruption is the maxillary canine. Other teeth that often fail to erupt as expected include the mandibular canine and maxillary and mandibular incisors and premolars.[1] All of these teeth may also be malpositioned and/or impacted. Table 6-1 shows the results of a study of 2,135 Air Force recruits selected at random.[2] Their panoramic radiographs revealed a certain frequency of impacted teeth (not including third molars):

Table 6-1.*

Canines:	0.9%	(0.7 maxillary, 0.2 mandibular)
Incisors:	0.17%	(all maxillary)
Premolars:	0.7%	(0.3 maxillary, 0.4 mandibular)
Molars:	0.5%	(0.4 maxillary, 0.1 mandibular)

*Because of the ages of participants in this study (approximately 18-20) it should be noted that some of them would already have received dental treatment for these conditions.

The content of this chapter is limited to a discussion of the "minor oral surgery/bonded bracket with fixed orthodontics" method of treating unerupted canines and incisors. Tooth attachment techniques (other than bonded brackets) which have been more commonly used in past years are still valuable and should be considered as possibilities available to the practitioner. They include uncovering and packing,[3] ligation chains,[4,5] friction pins,[6] metal crowns with or without eyelets,[7] plastic crowns[8] and castings or bands with lugs.[3,9,10] Although these methods may have merit in a given treatment situation, inherent complications such as tooth dislodgement and tooth devitalization make them less desirable than bonded brackets. In addition, it is usually easier and more convenient to use bonded brackets. Figure 6-1 illustrates several of the older ways.

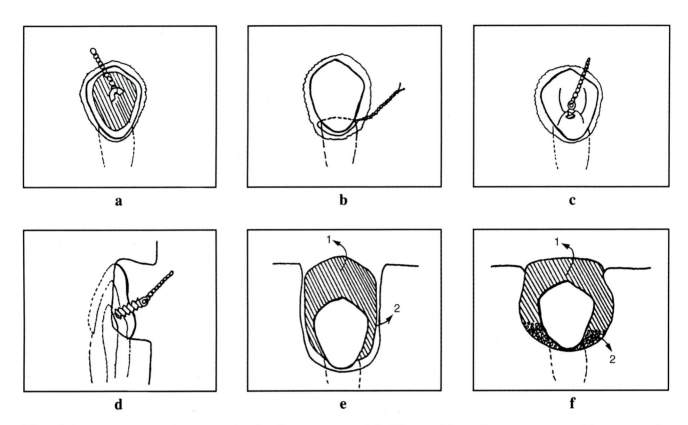

Fig. 6-1. a, A cemented cap. **b**, A wire ligature. **c and d**, The position of a screw tapped into a tooth. **e**, A plastic or metal crown cemented (2) and with zinc oxide-eugenol (ZOE) (1). **f**, The tooth is packed open for eruption with ZOE (1) and a gingival packing string (2). From Goodsell JF. Surgical exposure and orthodontic guidance of the impacted tooth. *Dent Clin N Am*. 1979; 23(3):385-392.

The surgical/orthodontic procedures described in this chapter are normally associated with full banding or bracketing of other teeth in the arch. However, if an unerupted tooth is the only orthodontic need of the patient and sufficient space exists for it to come into position, then the use of 2x6 bonded brackets (bonding of six anterior teeth along with bonding or banding both permanent first molars in either the maxillary or mandibular arch) will generally suffice.[11]

One of the main considerations with this procedure is the preservation of facial attached gingiva. When exposing unerupted teeth on the palate, this is not an issue since palatal mucosa is all of the attached variety; however, with labially positioned teeth the operator must always keep this thought in mind. This chapter presents examples of how teeth may be accessed and brought into the arch. Each differs somewhat from the other. There is usually not "just one method" to use in treating a given case. The approach will depend on tooth position, input from the person providing orthodontic treatment, and knowledge and experience of the surgeon.

Position and Timing

To localize the exact position of the tooth, the operator should use dual periapical radiographs and the buccal object rule. An occlusal film is also helpful to confirm the diagnosis. Panoramic films are not as precise in their value but will aid in providing supplemental information. Sometimes the tooth can be palpated.

As far as surgical timing is concerned, the tooth can be exposed and bracketed as soon as it is felt that it will not erupt on its own. This decision can generally be made six months to one year after the tooth would normally have erupted into the mouth.[12] At this time, the dentist is able to combine orthodontic traction forces with some remaining normal eruptive forces of the tooth.[13] For patient management, good local anesthesia and preferably some type of sedation (oral or intravenous) is desirable, especially when the procedure will be lengthy.

Maxillary Canines

When an unerupted canine is observed at a point in time beyond the normal period of eruption, an assessment is needed to determine the best of several possible treatment options. If possible, the dentist should try to prevent the need for any surgical intervention with these teeth. This can often be done with the early implementation of interceptive orthodontic methods. If, however, the conservative approach is not successful, surgery may be necessary.

Occasionally, the patient will present with a permanent canine that is either missing or so ectopically located that it cannot be brought into its normal position in the arch. It may be located either labially or lingually. Occasionally, an ectopic canine may be located so far from where it is needed that it should be removed or, in rare instances, subjected to long-term observation.[14] If retained, the operator should monitor changes such as cyst formation or pressure resorption of adjacent roots. Ectopic locations include close proximity to the nasal cavity and the maxillary sinus.

In this situation, the operator would consider:

1. keeping the deciduous canine (if it has sufficient root length and is esthetically acceptable),
2. establishment or maintenance of an incisor-premolar contact, or
3. fabrication of a prosthetic device.

If it is felt the tooth can be utilized, then another choice is surgical exposure followed by forced orthodontic extrusion. To accomplish this latter option, several methods are described in dental literature using both fixed and removable appliances.[4,15-19] They usually require the acquisition of additional space since the deciduous canine is smaller than its permanent successor.

SURGICAL TREATMENT

Maxillary Labial

Figure 6-2 (from the dental literature) depicts the use of a full-thickness trapezoidal flap apically repositioned and sutured in the new location. Note the author's emphasis on preservation of attached gingiva.

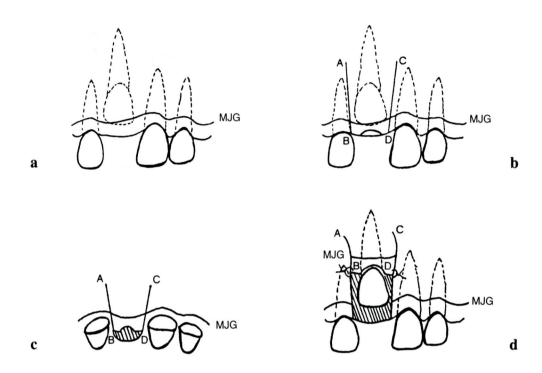

Fig. 6-2. Method for uncovering a tooth surgically without the loss of the attached gingiva. **a,** An unerupted tooth. **b,** A labial view of the incisor for flap design. The incision is from a to b and from c to d. **c,** An incisal view with points b and c connected and the shaded area removed. **d,** The flap has been pushed back and the attached gingival portion sutured into place. From Goodsell JF. Surgical exposure and orthodontic guidance of the impacted tooth. *Dent Clin N Am.* 1979; 23(3):385-392.

Figure 6-3 shows the result of a simple semilunar incision with flap reflection and apical repositioning. Suture placement is optional; they were not used in this instance. The semilunar incision was made with its apogee coronal to the level of the crown in attached gingiva. After the procedure, the attached tissue was immediately apical to the crown and accompanied the tooth as it was brought into alignment in the arch.

Originally, the tooth's labial surface was covered with alveolar mucosa. Merely making a window over the crown and positioning a bracket would not have been satisfactory since it probably would not have resulted in a collar of attached tissue.

Fig. 6-3, a. Preoperative photograph of a 13-year-old girl whose orthodontic treatment is on hold because of the canine's delayed eruption.

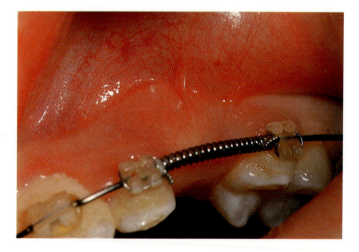

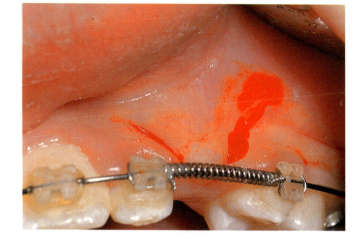

Fig. 6-3, b. Semilunar incision with its apogee well into attached gingiva.

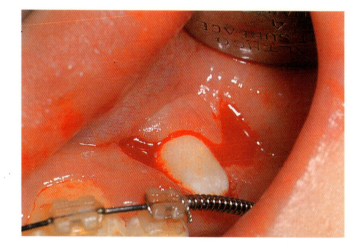

Fig. 6-3, c. Apical repositioning of a full-thickness mucoperiosteal flap. Flap length is assimilated into the flexibility of the mucobuccal fold. There is a limit to which this can be accomplished, but in this case it did not present a problem.

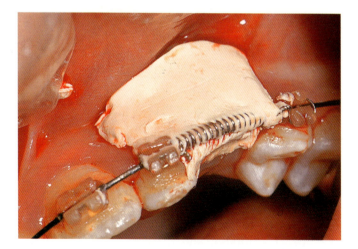

Fig. 6-3, d. Pack placement to protect the wound and stabilize the flap.

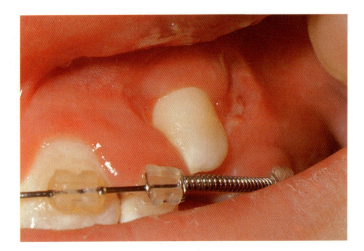

Fig. 6-3, e. Five-day postoperative view. A bracket may now be placed on the tooth.

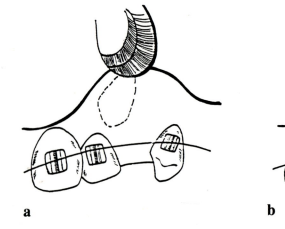

a

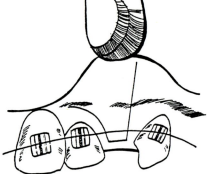

b

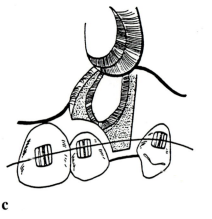

c

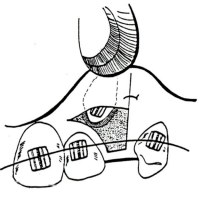

d

Fig. 6-4. In some cases, the operator may feel that there is too much tissue to reposition apically. **a-d** illustrates the technique for a laterally positioned flap that (1) exposes a sufficiently large segment of the tooth for bracket placement, (2) repositions some of the tissue that was over the tooth into the buccal vestibule, and (3) preserves a collar of attached gingiva in the appropriate place.

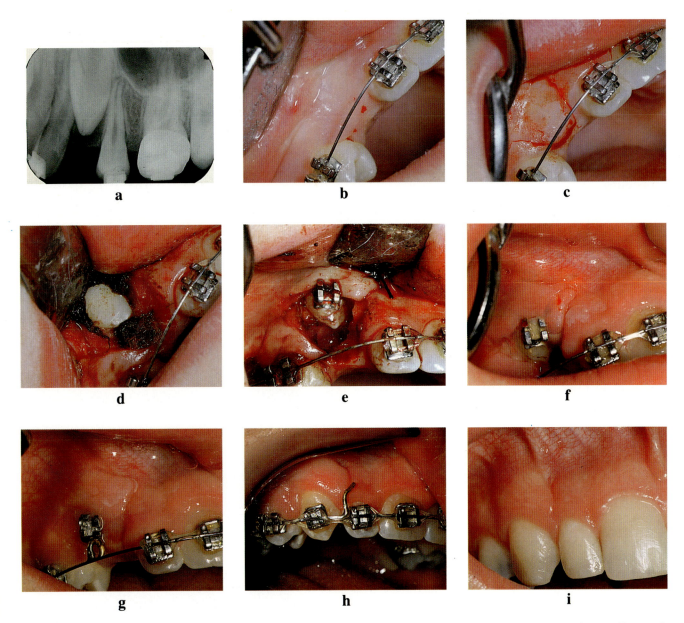

Fig. 6-5. This clinical case closely resembles the drawings from Figure 6-4. **a,** Preoperative radiograph showing a maxillary canine of a 13-year-old girl. **b,** Preoperative clinical view. **c,** Incision. The original intent of the operator was to apically reposition the flap in a manner similar to that used in Figure 6-1. When it was realized that there was too much tissue to accomplish this (the mucobuccal fold would not accommodate that much soft tissue), the operator chose to laterally position the flap. **d,** Tooth prepared for bracket placement. **e,** Bracket bonded and flap laterally positioned. **f,** Five-day postoperative healing. **g,** Two weeks postop. **h,** Four months postop. **i,** Eight months postop.

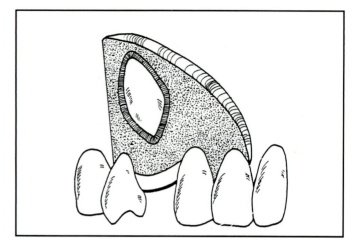

Fig. 6-6. Still another method of treatment is to uncover a tooth, bond a bracket to it, replace the flap in its original position, and then apply traction to the tooth by means of a ligature wire or gold chain attached to the bracket. **a.** This drawing illustrates the type of flap design that lends itself to this kind of procedure.

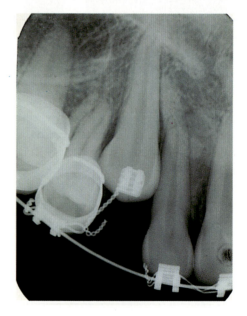

Fig. 6-6, b. Case in point. A submerged tooth is being pulled toward the archwire.

Fig. 6-6, c. Radiograph of the patient in **b.**

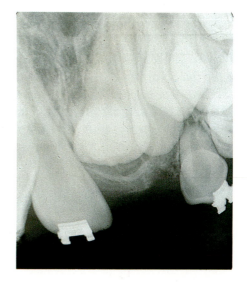

Fig. 6-7. This case shows the surgical technique for an unerupted maxillary incisor positioned facially and superiorly. Two teeth are to be uncovered, re-covered, and brought through tissue to the archwire. Periapical x-ray reveals unerupted teeth, including a supernumerary incisor.

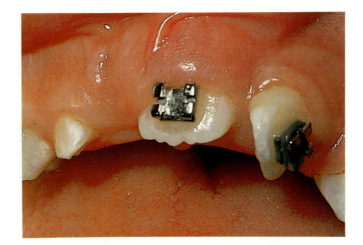

Fig. 6-8. Preoperative clinical view. One central incisor has failed to erupt in what is thought to be a normal period of time.

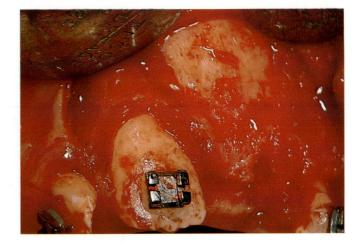

Fig. 6-9. *Step 1.* Reflect a full-thickness mucoperiosteal triangular flap exposing bone overlying the teeth. Later this flap will be repositioned to the same location. **Note:** Some operators will excise an ellipse of attached tissue at the crest of the ridge where the desired eruption will take place.

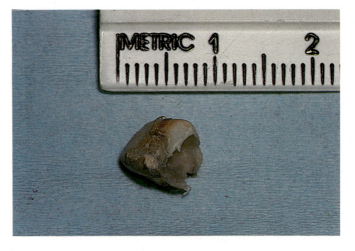

Fig. 6-10. *Step 2.* Remove bone, if necessary, to expose the facial surface of the tooth or teeth being bracketed. Remove the follicular covering of the tooth to be bracketed. Surgically remove any existing supernumerary teeth. A slow-speed handpiece bur is preferable to a high-speed one since it is less likely to inadvertently cut enamel.

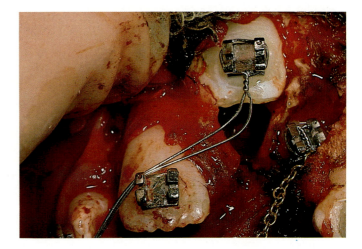

Fig. 6-11. Obtain hemostasis with local anesthetic containing 1:50,000 epinephrine and desired hemostatic agents, then pumice, dry, etch, and bond the bracket. Bond the bracket to the middle third of the tooth if possible. Fastening the ligation wire to the bracket before bonding seems to make initial arch wire attachment easier.

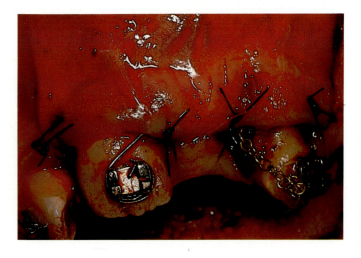

Fig. 6-12. *Step 3.* Reposition the full-thickness flap and suture. Eruption to normal position in the arch usually takes 6-12 months of orthodontic treatment.[1]

Figures 6-13 through 6-17 show postoperative healing at five days, five months, six months, seven months, and eight months. Figure 6-16 shows an absence of attached gingiva that gave the dentist reason for concern over the ultimate prognosis of the case. When the central incisor was brought into the arch, however, these concerns were alleviated as the tooth demonstrated a generous band of attached tissue. It is believed that this regenerated gingiva is derived from the periodontal ligament.[20]

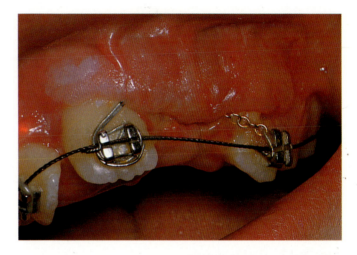

Fig. 6-13. Five days.

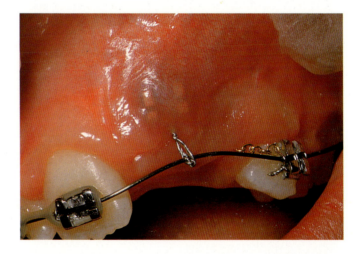

Fig. 6-14. Five months.

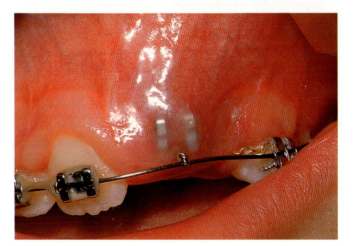

Fig. 6-15. Six months.

Fig. 6-16. Seven months.

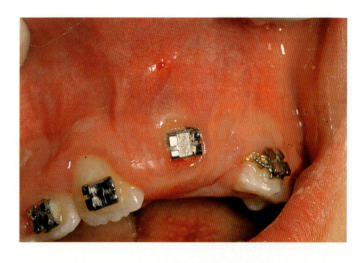

Fig. 6-17. Eight months.

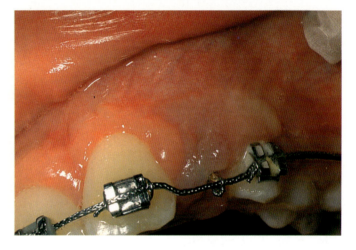

Maxillary Lingual

The following section describes methods to consider in dealing with anterior unerupted teeth located on the palatal side of the arch.

Superficially positioned teeth:

1. Create a surgical window in the palatal mucosa and remove bone to expose the enamel. To place a metal or plastic crown on the unerupted tooth (a technique not commonly used in recent times), it is suggested that a two millimeter wide groove be made around the entire crown and that the tooth be mildly luxated to allow the crown to slip into place.[13] For bracket placement, much less bone needs to be removed and the tooth never needs luxation.

2. Establish hemostasis and then polish, dry, and etch the tooth.

3. Place the bracket. If the tooth is rotated, it may be necessary to rebracket once the tooth gets closer to its final position.

4. Attach the ligature wire to the arch wire with light pressure.

Deeply embedded teeth:

1. Expose the enamel surface of the tooth by reflecting a palatal full-thickness mucoperiosteal flap.
2. Create a channel in the bone along the expected pathway that the tooth will take to its final position.
3. Follow steps 2, 3, and 4, as described on previous page for superficially positioned teeth.
4. Reposition the flap.

Table 6-2. Bracketing Unerupted Tooth Flowchart

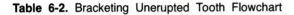

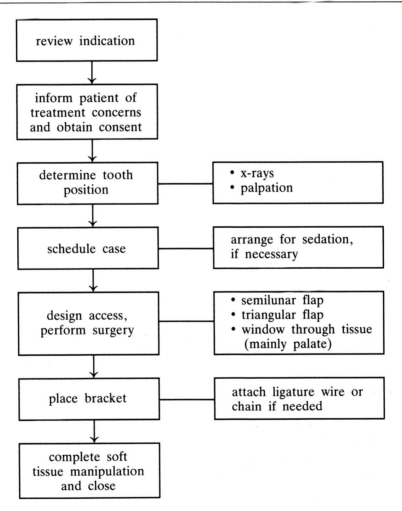

CLINICAL CASE

Case 1

Full-Thickness Flap Reflection Followed by Bracketing and Flap Replacement

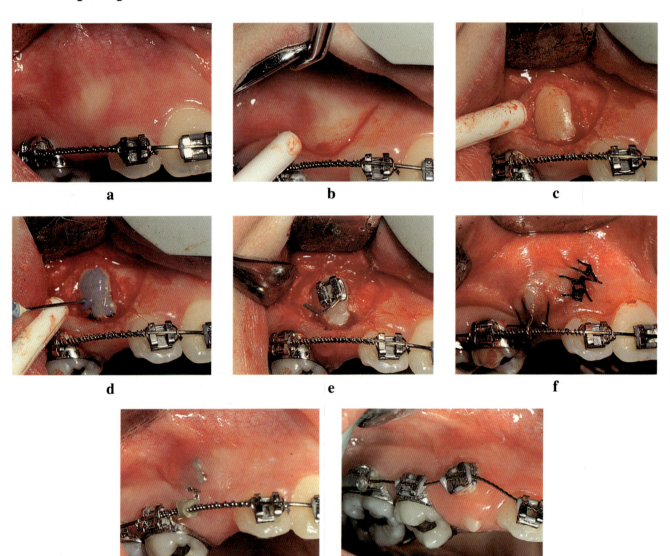

Fig. 6-18 a, Facial enamel of an unerupted canine can be seen through translucent gingival tissue. The tooth is delayed in its eruption. **b,** Semilunar incision for the subsequent full-thickness flap. **c,** Flap reflection—tooth exposed. In retrospect, the most coronal aspect of the incision should have been closer to the ridge crest since the flap, when repositioned, will have a portion of the incision line resting on enamel, not bone. **d,** The tooth is dried and then etched. **e,** The bracket is bonded to the tooth. **f,** Tissue replaced and sutured. Part of the suture line is at risk for dehiscence. **g,** Two week postop. Healing is progressing and the bracket is ready to emerge through tissue. The coronal part of the flap exceeded expectations and healed normally. **h,** Two months postop.

References

1. Shapira Y, Mischler WA, and Kuftince MM. The displaced mandibular canine. *J Dent Child*. 1982;49:362.

2. Langenderfer WR et al. An analysis of pantomographs from U.S. Air Force recruits. *General Dentistry*. May-June, 1985;224.

3. Lewis PD. Preorthodontic surgery in the treatment of the impacted canines. *Am J Orthod*. 1971;60:382.

4. Goodsell JF. Surgical exposure and orthodontic guidance of the impacted tooth. *Den Clin N Am*. 1979;23(3):385.

5. Revell JH. Surgical orthodontics. *Int J Orthod*. 1964;2:5.

6. Prescott M, and Goldberg M. Controlled eruption of impacted teeth with threaded pins. *J Oral Surg*. 1969;27(8):615.

7. Laskin DM, and Peskins S. Surgical aids in orthodontics. *Dent Clin North Am*. July, 1968;p.509.

8. Clark D. The management of impacted canines – free physiologic eruption. *J Am Orthod*. 1971;82:836.

9. Kettle MA. Treatment of the unerupted maxillary canine. *Dent Pract*. 1958;8:245.

10. Johnston WD. Treatment of palatally impacted canine teeth. *Am J Orthod*. 1969;56:589.

11. Sim JM. *Minor Tooth Movement in Children*, ed. 2. St. Louis, Mo: CV Mosby Co. 1977;96.

12. McKay C. Unerupted maxillary canine: assessment of the role of surgery in 2500 treated cases. *Br Dent J*. 1978;145:207.

13. Laskin DM. *Oral and Maxillofacial Surgery*, vol 2. St. Louis, Mo: CV Mosby Co. 1985;101.

14. Alling CC. Impacted canine teeth. *Dental Clin North Am*. 1979;23(3):439.

15. Fifield CA. Surgery and orthodontic treatment for unerupted teeth. *JADA*. 1986;113:590.

16. McDonald F, and Yap WL. The surgical exposure and application of direct traction of unerupted teeth. *Am J Orthod*. 1979;89(4):331.

17. Hunt NP. Direct traction applied to the unerupted teeth using acid-etch technique. *Br J Orthod*. 1977;5:211.

18. Barnett DP, and Leonard MS. A simple method of applying traction to buried teeth. *Dent Update*. 1976;3:8.

19. Genisor AM, and Strauss RE. The direct bonding technique applied to the management of the maxillary impacted canine. *J Am Dent Assoc*. 1974;89:1332.

20. Lundberg M, and Wennstrom JL. Development of gingiva following surgical exposure of a facially positioned unerupted incisor. *J Perio*. 1988;652.

Additional Reading Material

1. Andreasen GF. A review of approaches to treatment of impacted maxillary cuspids. *Oral Surg*. 1971;31:479.

2. Bass TB. Observations of the misplaced upper canine tooth. *Dent Pract*. 1976;18:25.

3. Boyd RL. Clinical assessment of injuries in orthodontic movement of impacted teeth. I. Methods of attachment. *Am J Orthod*. 1982;82:478.

4. Geiger AM. A simple technique for management of the high palatally impacted canine. *J Oral Maxillofac Surg*. 1987;45:643.

5. Hardy P. The autogenous transplantation of maxillary canines. *Br Dent J*. 1982;153:183.

6. Heaney TG, and Atherton JD. Periodontal problems associated with the surgical exposure of unerupted teeth. *Br J Orthod*. 1976;5:79.

7. Hunter SB. The treatment of the unerupted maxillary canine. Parts I and II. *Br Dent J*. 1983;154:294,335.

8. Shiloah J, and Kopczyk RA. Mucogingival considerations in surgical exposure of maxillary impacted canines. *J Dent Child*. 1978;45:79.

9. Wisth PJ, Norderval K, and Boe OE. Periodontal status of orthodontically treated impacted maxillary canines. *Angle Orthod*. 1976;46:69.

Chapter 7

Preserving Alveolar Ridge Contours With Synthetic Bone

Introduction
The Nature of Synthetic Bone
  Types of Synthetic Bone
  Particle Sizes
Alveolar Ridge Defects
  Clinical Considerations
Clinical Cases
  Treatment Flowchart

INTRODUCTION

When extracting teeth, be it one or several, it is not uncommon for facial and/or crestal alveolar bone to be lost because of either infection or traumatic exodontia. This may not matter a great deal in the posterior of the mouth, since appearance is usually secondary to function. A bridge pontic can be shaped to meet the ridge regardless of its height, and in the lower arch, sanitary bridges are acceptable. However, in the anterior, especially in a patient with a high smile line, it can result in serious esthetic concerns.

Rather than accepting normal healing following surgery and later having to consider a second surgical procedure to reestablish optimum ridge contours, it is usually better to place a bone graft in the post-extraction site, obtain primary (or near primary) closure over the material, and then anticipate healing that will preserve the ridge's normal configuration. A few months later, a bridge may be fabricated with the pontic approximating the ridge in an ideal manner.

If the intrasurgical opportunity is missed, then there may be no choice but to resort to a second surgery to enhance a resorbed alveolar ridge. This secondary surgical event could involve a soft tissue procedure (such as a connective tissue graft or repositioning of connective tissue) or an osseous procedure (such as a synthetic or natural bone graft for ridge augmentation) to increase ridge height, eliminate undercuts, or round out flat or negative contours.[1-5] In addition to their application in post-extraction sites, bone grafts can be applied in such limited-use situations as pathologic defects in alveolar bone, periodontal infrabony pockets, and subperiosteally to help stabilize the hypermobile ridge for dentures.

This writing emphasizes the use of synthetic bone, realizing that natural bone (autogenous or freeze-dried grafts) may be more applicable in some circumstances. The disadvantages of autografts (from one place to another in the same individual) are accessibility and the discomfort of a second surgery site. The main disadvantage of allografts, formerly called homografts (from one member of the species to another, such as freeze-dried bone) is the cost. Most types of synthetic bone are biocompatible and relatively inexpensive.

THE NATURE OF SYNTHETIC BONE

Types of Synthetic Bone

Five different synthetic bone materials are currently available:

1. Dense, ceramic hydroxyapatite . . . . nonresorbable

2. Porous (beta) tricalcium phosphate . . . . resorbable

3. Replamineform hydroxyapatite . . . . nonresorbable

4. Porous polymethylmethacrylate resin . . . . nonresorbable

5. Non-ceramic, pure hydroxyapatite . . . . resorbable

Hydroxyapatite (also referred to as hydroxylapatite or durapatite) has been successfully tested for biocompatibility.[6-10] Hydroxyapatite is osteoconductive rather than osteoinductive, in that when implanted to an area where bone is normally found, it serves as a scaffold within which host tissues deposit new bone peripherally, but when implanted into an area where bone is not normally found, it becomes encapsulated within a connective tissue stroma. It does not induce the formation of bone or cementum.[6,11] In alveolar bone ridge sites, it merely acts as a biocompatible foreign-body filler.

The inorganic phase of human mineralized tissue is derived from the calcium phosphate system. With the discovery of advanced sintering techniques in the late 1960's, calcium phosphate salts were produced in a ceramic form.[12-14] Sintering is a process by which individual tricalcium phosphate ($Ca_3[PO_4]2$) or hydroxyapatite ($Ca10[PO_4]6[OH]2$) crystals are first compressed and then heated to 1,100 - 1,300 degrees Centigrade. This allows the crystals to fuse at the crystal-grain boundaries, forming a dense ceramic material.[8]

Particle shapes include spherical, multifaceted and irregular. It is not clear which, if any, are most conducive to clinical success.[15]

Porous (beta) tricalcium phosphate has been demonstrated to be biocompatible,[16-18] bioresorbable,[19,20] and has osteoconductive properties. It is felt by some researchers that tricalcium phosphate particles have to be resorbed before new bone can be formed, thus delaying the healing process somewhat.[21,22] It is suggested that it is a nidus for new bone formation and not merely an inert filler.[23] Once the graft has been transformed into newly formed bone, implants may be placed in the area.

Replamineform hydroxyapatite. It is difficult for modern technology to produce ceramic materials with a porosity similar to bone; however, such a structure does exist in one species of marine coral (porites). When this substance is formulated so that it can be used clinically, it is known as replamineform hydroxyapatite.

Porous replamineform hydroxyapatite is biocompatible and is reported to allow bone ingrowth into its pores. It is slightly bioresorbable,[8,24] one percent per year, beginning about twelve months postoperatively.[25] It seems to possess superior osteoconductive properties, but lacks osteoinductive potential.[8] This is an excellent synthetic material because of uniform pore sizes, desirable chemical composition, and scaffold-like qualities that promote the ingrowth and formation of new bone tissue in osseous defects.

When this material is compared to dense HA in ridge augmentation, there seems to be greater bone growth into the porous HA (replamineform) than into dense HA, but the difference is not statistically significant. At six months, most bone growth that will occur from the underlying alveolar bone has already occurred.

Porous polymethylmethacrylate resin (a polymer — HTR or "hard tissue replacement") is a composite of biocompatible materials that encourages bone growth by creating a nonresorbable, microscopic scaffolding into which new bone can grow. It is available in granular form or it can be molded at the operative site into a solid form. It is hydrophilic and electrically active – qualities that promote new bone formation.

Non-ceramic, pure hydroxyapatite is a resorbable graft material. It is nonceramic because it is not taken beyond the sintering point in the manufacturing process.

Particle Sizes

There are generally two uses for synthetic implant material produced by manufacturers, namely placement in periodontal pockets and in alveolar ridge defects not associated with teeth, such as post-extraction sites. Particle size is matched to desired use (Table 7-1).

Table 7-1. Synthetic Bone Particle Sizes

Alveolar ridge
- larger particles
- 10-40 mesh (particles 600-2000 micron width)
- surgical objectives:
    - –to reconstruct atrophic edentulous alveolar ridges
    - –to restore stability of hypermobile edentulous ridges

Periodontal pocket
- smaller particles
- 30-100 mesh (particles about 400-600 micron width)
    - Note: mesh size is inversely proportional to microns
- surgical objectives:
    - –to restore periodontal osseous defects
    - –to improve ridge contour and esthetics

Prior to using synthetic bone, the operator should determine the use for which it is intended and then settle on one or more types to have on hand.

ALVEOLAR RIDGE DEFECTS

Clinical Considerations

Using synthetic bone particles to augment osseous defects has definite clinical advantages. The material maintains ridge form for esthetic appearance and prevents the collapse of overlying gingival tissue. It is easy to obtain, inexpensive, and generally a covered benefit of insurance carriers. This operation may not be indicated for all patients, but it is an alternative to subsequent soft tissue or osseous grafting procedures.[26]

These bone grafts can be combined with different types of postoperative restorative choices such as fixed bridgework (acid-etched or conventional bridges) or removable prosthetics.

Success is ensured with:
- careful flap reflection
- thorough debridement of the wound

- profuse saline irrigation
- careful handling of the graft material
- proper suturing
- a protective dressing to stabilize and protect the material during clot formation
- systemic antibiotics
- attention to asepsis

It is not unusual for some particles to exfoliate through granulating tissue or maturing epithelium during the first 2-3 weeks after surgery. Postoperative care includes frequent checkups to monitor healing and help prevent or treat problems such as infection.

CLINICAL CASES
Case 1
Synthetic Bone in an Extraction Site Ravaged By Infection, Followed by a Bridge

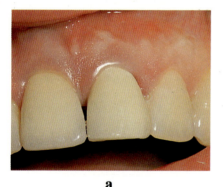
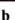
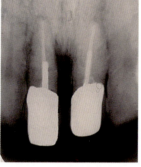
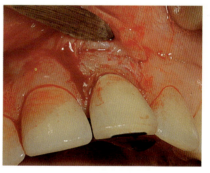

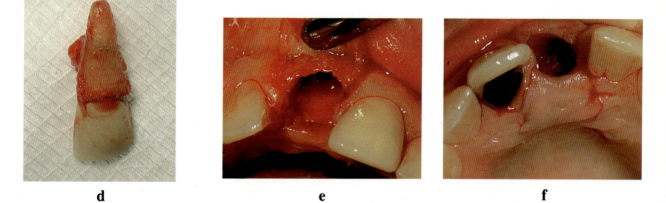

a   b   c

d   e   f

Fig. 7-1. a, The patient's right central, originally injured in a traumatic accident, has been treated endodontically and crowned. It is now being rejected by the body through gradual avulsion. It has a nine millimeter pocket and purulent exudate that emanates from the sulcus. There has been considerable loss of alveolar bone. **b,** Radiographic view. **c,** Since the placement of synthetic bone is anticipated, releasing incisions are made to help accomplish more complete postoperative closure. **d,** Offending tooth. **e,** Extraction site. **f,** Lingual view.

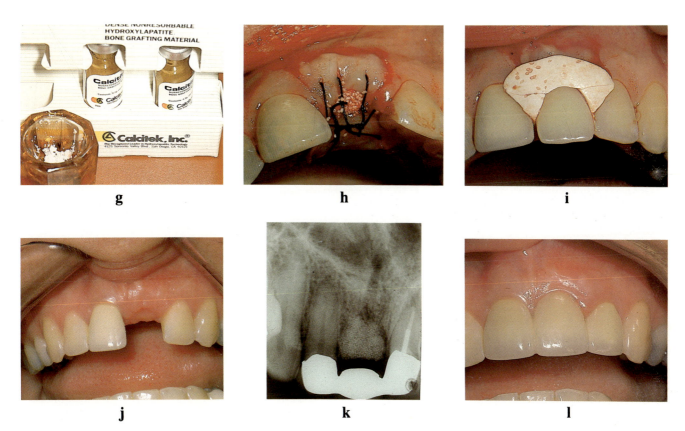

Fig. 7-1 cont. g, Nonresorbable particulate material placed to help maintain optimum ridge contours. **h,** Closure. **i,** Periopack (under flipper partial) helps maintain the surface blood clot and prevent the loss of particles. **j,** Two-week postoperative healing. **k,** Radiographic view after bridge placement. **l,** Final restoration.

Case 2
Result of Labial Plate Loss
Without Augmentation

Fig. 7-2. When this patient's lateral incisor was removed, there was extensive labial bone loss. This 70-year-old individual rejected treatment with a second surgery to restore normal ridge contour. The new pontic attempts to satisfy esthetic and functional requirements in a compromised situation.

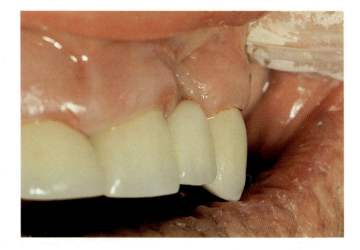

Case 3
Synthetic Bone Placement Followed by Single Tooth Implant

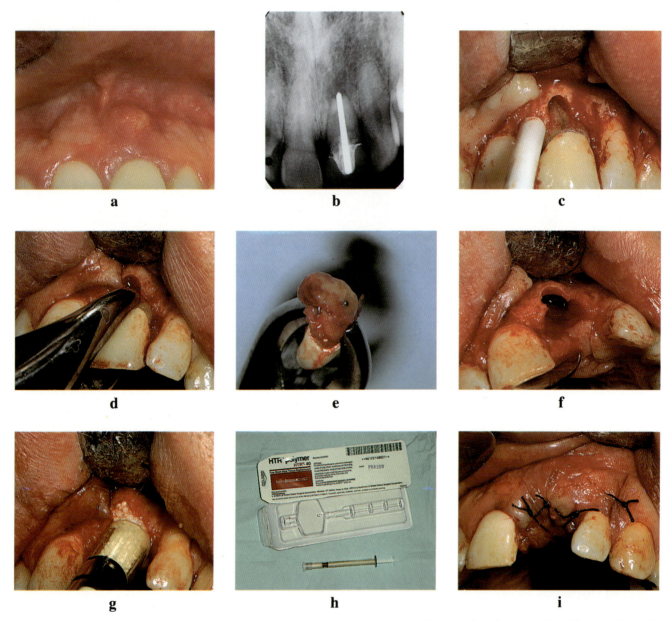

Fig. 7-3. a, Clinical appearance of a periapical abscess. **b,** Radiographic view of the diseased tooth showing an overextended post. **c,** Flap retraction revealing a vertical root fracture. **d,** Extraction. **e,** Periapical view of the extracted tooth. **f,** Socket. **g,** Nonresorbable synthetic bone being placed in the socket by use of a syringe. **h,** Synthetic bone material. **i,** Closure.

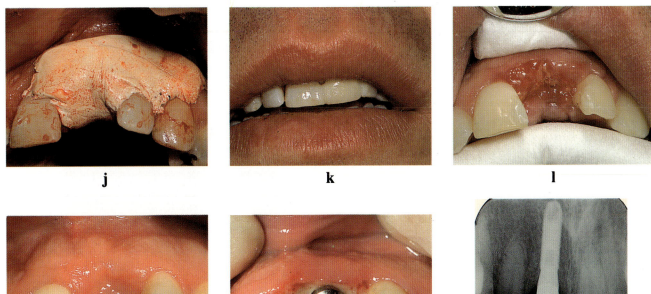

j   k   l

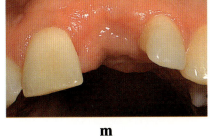

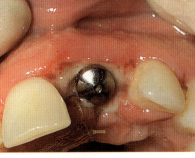

m   n   o

Fig. 7-3 cont, **j,** Wound covered with periopack. **k,** The patient's own crown was cut from the root and bonded into position to serve provisionally until a flipper partial can be fabricated and inserted. **l,** One-week postoperative healing. **m,** Two-week healing. **n,** The patient consulted an oral surgeon and agreed to a single-tooth implant. The implant was placed through and apically beyond the synthetic material. If the implant had been anticipated, resorbable bone particles would have been used. **o,** Radiograph of implant. **p,** Single tooth restoration on the implant. Follow-up surgery is scheduled to refine gingival adaptation.

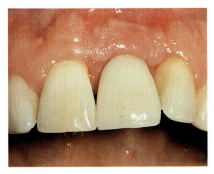

p

Case 4
Synthetic Bone Placement Followed By Maryland Bridge

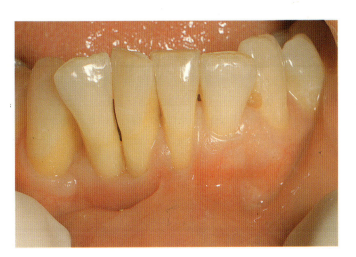

Fig. 7-4, a. This 45-year-old woman has two incisors (teeth #'s 25 and 26) that have severe periodontitis and are symptomatic.

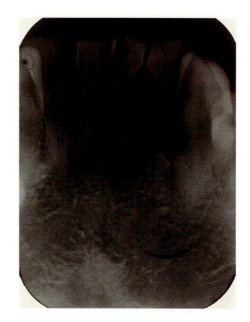

Fig. 7-4, b. Chronic infection has eroded bone from around the roots.

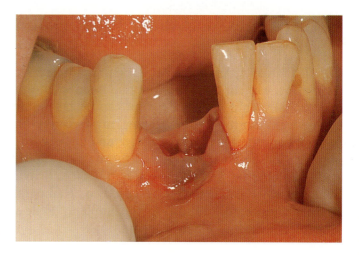

Fig. 7-4, c. The teeth were extracted.

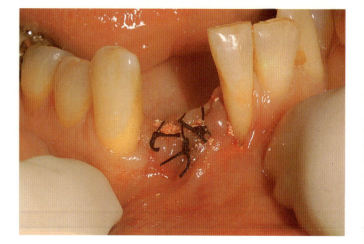

Fig. 7-4, d. Synthetic bone was inserted into the sockets to help maintain as much ridge height as possible.

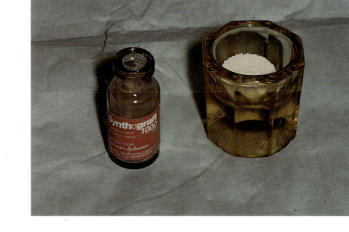

Fig. 7-4, e. Tricalcium phosphate (resorbable) synthetic bone that was used.

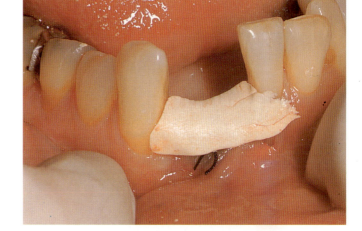

Fig. 7-4, f. Wound covered with periopack.

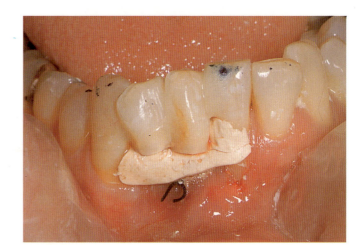

Fig. 7-4, g. The patient's own teeth (crowns) were used as temporaries.

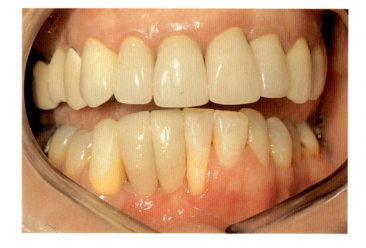

Fig. 7-4, h. Postoperative healing.

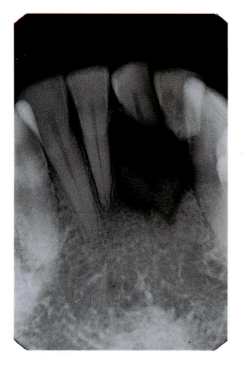

Fig. 7-4, i. Postoperative radiograph.

Fig. 7-4, j. Maryland bridge placed two months postoperatively, double-abutted on each side.

Case 5
Synthetic Bone Placement in Two Sockets Followed by a Bridge

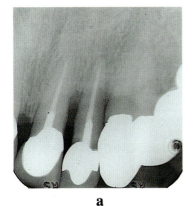

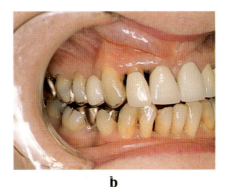

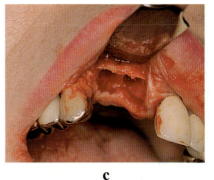

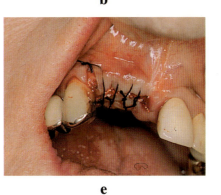

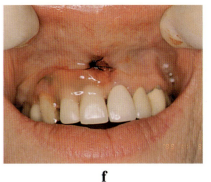

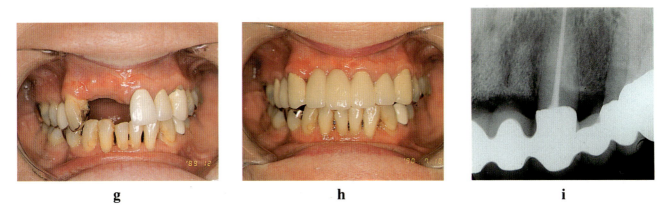

Fig. 7-5. a, Initial radiograph of #7 and #8 showing advanced periodontitis. **b**, Preoperative picture revealing severe osseous and gingival recession of #7 and #8 along with a poor esthetic situation. **c**, Buccal flap reflection with vertical incision at the distal to facilitate atraumatic extraction of #7 and #8 and thorough debridement of the sockets. There is paper-thin labial bone, no interseptal bone, and susceptibility to continued resorption rather than repair. **d**, Extraction defect filled with nonresorbable hydroxyapatite. **e**, Primary closure should be attempted. The closer buccal and labial sides are approximated, the fewer particles will be lost and the easier and faster re-epithelialization will take place. **f**, A maxillary flipper partial is placed for the temporary replacement of #7 and #8. A light-cured, gingival-colored periodontal packing material is placed as a protective dressing over the wound for 5-7 days. **g**, The healed ridge at approximately 6 weeks postextraction shows good contours. **h**, This picture shows the final restoration 8 months postoperatively. **i**, Radiograph at 8 months posttreatment. Tooth #6 has had endodontic therapy.

Table 7-2. Synthetic bone flowchart

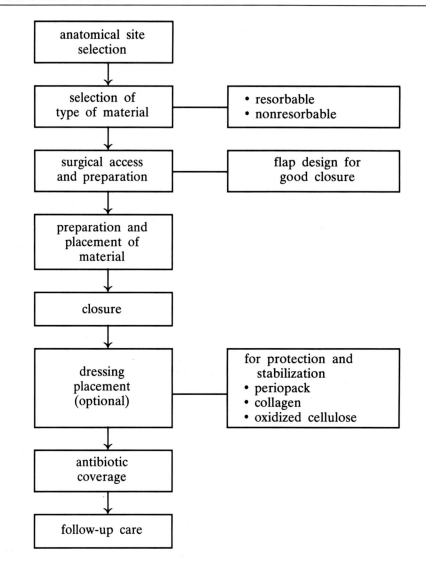

References

1. Boyne PJ et al. Long term study of hydroxylapatite implants in canine alveolar bone. *J Oral Maxillofac Surg.* 1984;42:589.

2. Kent J et al. Correction of alveolar ridge deficiencies with nonresorbable hydroxyapatite. *J Am Dent Assoc.* 1982;105(6):993.

3. Fox WD, Dolan EA, and White JT. Hydroxylapatite augmentation of a maxillary defect. *Gen Dent.* 1985;May/June:248.

4. Cohen H. Localized ridge augmentation with hydroxylapatite report of case. *JADA.* 1984;108(1):54.

5. Kaminishi R et al. Reconstruction of alveolar width for orthodontic tooth movement: a case report. *Am J Orthod.* 1987;89(4)342.

6. Froum SJ et al. Human clinical and histologic responses to durapatite implants in intraosseous lesions: case reports. *J Perio.* 1982;53:714.

7. Misiek DJ et al. Soft tissue response to different shaped hydroxyapatite particles. *J Dent Res.* 1983;62:196.

8. Holmes RE. Bone regeneration within a coralline hydroxyapatite implant. *Plast Reconstr Surg.* 1979;63:626.

9. Kent J et al. Alveolar ridge augmentation using non-resorbable hydroxyapatite with or without autogenous cancellous bone. *J Oral Maxillofac Surg*. 1983;41:629.

10. Nery EB et al. Functional loading of bioceramic-augmented alveolar ridge – a pilot study. *J Prosthet Dent*. 1975;43:338.

11. Moskow BS, Lubarr A. Histological assessment of human periodontal defect after Durapatite ceramic implant; Report of a case. *J Perio*. 1985;54:455.

12. Driskell TD, Hassler CR, and McCoy LR. The significance of resorbable bioceramics in the repair of bone defects. *Proc 26th Annual Conf Eng Med Biol*. 1973;15:199.

13. Hubbard WG, Hirthe WM, and Mueller KH. Physiological calcium phosphate implants. *Proc 26th Annual Conf Eng Med Biol*. 1973;15:198.

14. Monroe EX et al. New calcium phosphate ceramic material for bone and tooth implants. *J Dent Res*. 1971;50:860.

15. Association Report. Hydroxylapatite, beta tricalcium phosphate, and autogenous and allogenic bone for filling periodontal defects, alveolar ridge augmentation, and pulp capping. Council on Dental Materials, Instruments, and Equipment; Council on Dental Therapeutics, *JADA*. 1984;108:822.

16. Braly T. The use of Synthograft in periodontal bony defects. *J Oral Implant*. 1983;10(4):611-618.

17. Hoexter DL. The use of tricalcium phosphate (Synthograft). Its use in extensive periodontal defects. *J Oral Implan*. 1983;10(4):599-610.

18. Shen TC. Tricalcium phosphate (Synthograft) in a vital homogenous tooth transplant. *Gen Dent*.1985;November/ December: 518-519.

19. Bhaskar SN. Biodegradable ceramic implants in bone. *Oral Surg*. 1971;32:336.

20. Metsger DS, Driskell TD, and Paulsrud JR. Tri-calcium phosphate ceramic, a resorbable bone implant: review and current status. *J Am Dent Assoc*. 1982;105:1035.

21. Levin MP, Getter L, and Cutright DE. A comparison of iliac marrow and biodegradable ceramic in periodontal defects. *J Biomed Mater Res*. 1975:9:183.

22. Nery EB et al. Bioceramic implants in surgically produced infrabony defects. *J Perio*. 1978;46:523.

23. Bowers GM et al. Histologic observations following the placement of tricalcium implants in human intrabony defects. *J Perio*. 1986;57:286.

24. Finn RA, Bell WH, and Brammer JA. Interpositional "grafting" with autogenous bone and coralline hydroxyapatite. *J Maxillofac Surg*. 1980;8:217.

25. Piecuch JF et al. Experimental ridge augmentation with porous hydroxyapatite implants. *J Dent Res*. 1983;62:148.

26. Hoen MM et. al. Preserving the maxillary anterior alveolar ridge contour using hydroxylapatite. *JADA*. 1989;118:739-741.

Suggested Reading

1. Bowers GM. New attachment – fact or fallacy? Presented at the Midwest Periodontal Meeting, Chicago, February, 1985.

2. Hoexter DL, Minichetti JC. The use of durapatite ceramic implant in the treatment of juvenile periodontitis: a case report. *Comp Dent Ed*. July/August 1986;VII(7):458-466.

3. Krejci CB, Farah CF, and Bissada NF. Osseous grafting in periodontal therapy, Part I: osseous graft materials. *Compend Contin Educ Dent*. 1987;8(9):722-728.

4. Piecuch JF et al. Experimental ridge augmentation with porous hydroxyapatite implants. *J Dent Res*. 1983;62:148.

5. Piecuch JF. Extraskeletal implantation of porous hydroxyapatite ceramic. *J Dent Res*. 1982;61:1458.

6. Yukna RA. Practical periodontics in the 80s. Presented at the Fall meeting, Cleveland Academy of Advanced Dental Education. October, 1985.

Chapter 8

Management of the Abnormal Frenum

INTRODUCTION

Hypertrophic or malpositioned frenae frequently present problems in dental treatment. These difficulties may be in patients who are young or old, dentulous or edentulous. They exist in anterior or posterior regions of the mouth and in maxillary or mandibular arches. On the lower arch, they can be on the facial or lingual sides of the ridge.

The frenum consists of epithelium, connective tissue, nerves, and occasionally fat and muscle tissue. Elastic fibers are found traversing the entire length of the frenum, beginning at their insertion in the periosteum. In most cases, the frenum terminates close to the mucogingival line. When a facial frenum projects nearer the ridge crest, exerting traction on lingual tissues or on sulcular epithelium, there can be adverse effects on the periodontium.

Problems with frenum attachments concern many disciplines of dentistry, impacting on orthodontic, periodontic, restorative and prosthetic treatments.

Although there is some disagreement on what constitutes a "normal" frenum, there is a general consensus on what constitutes one that is pathologic. The following descriptions help identify an undesirable anatomic situation:

- close proximity to the interdental gingival margin
- greater than normal width in attached gingiva
- blanching of the interdental and/or palatal tissues when the lip is stretched

Table 8-1. The Interdisciplinary Significance of Frenae

Discipline	Problem	Comment
Orthodontics	Midline diastema. Abnormal maxillary labial frenum.	Frenectomy and fiberotomy after space closure.
Prosthodontics	Esthetics in anterior.	Removal of large, fleshy frenum in patients with high lip line improves esthetics.
	Denture retention.	Abnormal frenum displaces denture, reduces stability.
Oral surgery	Need for frenectomy or vestibuloplasty.	For enhancement of denture with improved retention, esthetics.
Periodontics	Gingival margin integrity.	Tension from frenum detaches marginal tissue.
	Gingival stability after treatment.	Tension from frenum inhibits soft tissue reattachment.
	Attached gingiva.	Abnormal frenum diminishes or prevents adequate zone of attached gingiva.
	Plaque control.	Abnormal frenum attachment inhibits adequate plaque control.

MAXILLARY LABIAL FRENUM

Diagnostic Criteria

The maxillary labial frenum is a remnant of an embryonic structure that connected the tubercle of the upper lip to the palatine papilla. As the alveolar process grows vertically, the frenum usually reattaches more apically. The failure of attached frenal fibers to migrate apically results in a residual band of tissue between the maxillary central incisors which has been considered as an important causative factor in persistent or relapsed midline diastemas.

A midline diastema may be the result of an aberrant frenum, but the frenum is generally not the only cause. Midline diastemas are normal for most seven to eight-year-olds, but by age eighteen, only seven percent of those diastemas remain. While a classic study by Edwards[1] found a positive correlation between the presence of abnormal frenae and diastemas, it was also found:

- many diastemas were associated with normal frenae
- many subjects with abnormal frenae had no diastema
- many diastemas which were orthodontically closed relapsed even when a normal frenum was present
- some subjects had relapse of orthodontically treated diastemas even when the frenum was treated surgically

The relationship between the abnormal frenum and the midline diastema presents a strong, but not absolute, correlation. Other etiologic factors for midline diastema must be considered as well, including:

1. Improper axial inclination of the roots
2. Tooth size discrepancies
3. Pernicious habits (thumb, finger, lip, tongue, etc.)
4. Deleterious occlusal patterns, contacts
5. Tooth anatomy (wider cervically than incisally)
6. Muscular imbalances
7. Supernumerary teeth

There is some disagreement between orthodontic and oral surgery literature on the timing of surgical treatment involving the frenum. Some oral surgery literature advocates procedures for frenum excision prior to the closure of the diastema. This can, however, lead to the undesirable and unesthetic loss of interproximal tissue. There is presently a consensus among dental clinicians that treatment of the frenum is most clinically valid after the eruption of all six permanent anterior teeth has failed to close the diastema – and then in conjunction with active orthodontic treatment. This seems to provide a more stable and definitely more esthetic result.

Placek, Skach and Mrklas[2] established a clinical classification of the maxillary labial frenum to provide guidelines for treatment.

Table 8-2.

Frenum Type	Level of frenum attachment	
Mucosal	attachment at the mucogingival junction	(Fig. 8-1)
Gingival	attachment to attached gingiva	(Fig. 8-2)
Papillary	attachment to the interdental papilla	(Fig. 8-3)
Papillary penetrating	attached to the interdental papilla but penetrating through to the incisive papilla	(Fig. 8-4)

The two papillary types of attachment are regarded as pathological and potentially problematic.

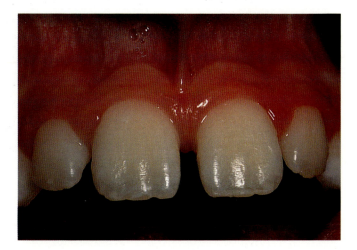

Fig. 8-1. Mucosal attachment.

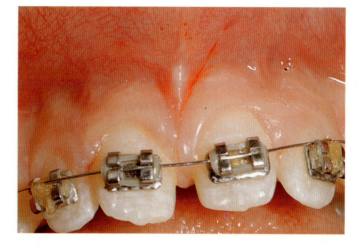

Fig. 8-2. Gingival attachment.

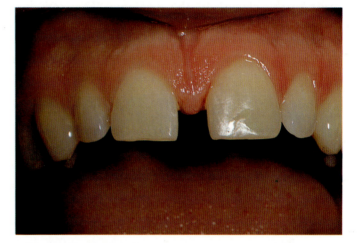

Fig. 8-3. Papillary attachment.

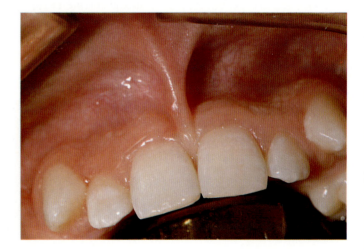

Fig. 8-4. Papillary penetrating attachment.

Surgical Treatment of the Maxillary Labial Frenum: Frenotomy

Frenotomy involves the partial removal of the frenum using incisions in mucosal tissue only. Periosteum is not affected. The frenum may also be repositioned.

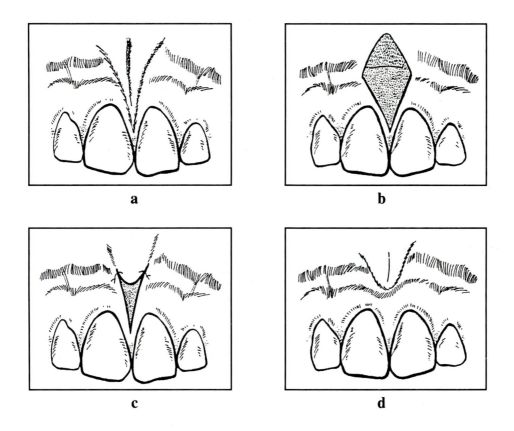

Fig. 8-5. a, Frenum attached to the interdental papilla. **b,** Incisions made parallel to the lateral borders of the frenum. As the frenum is undermined, gentle tension on the frenum allows access to dissect it apically and laterally from underlying connective tissue. **c,** The flap containing the frenum is apically relocated at or above the mucogingival line and sutured. **d,** Healing produces a frenum which has been relocated apically with a corresponding increase in the zone of attached gingival tissue labial to the central incisors.

Z-Plasty

Z-Plasty is a type of frenotomy that only requires incisions in alveolar mucosa. Periosteum is undisturbed. It involves a shifting of two mucosal flaps, thereby changing the tissue fiber direction from vertical to near horizontal.

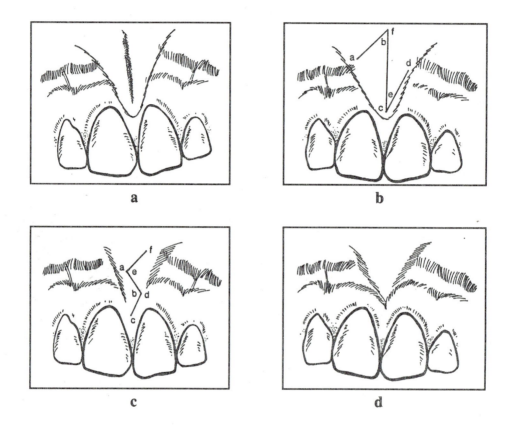

a   b

c   d

Fig. 8-6. a, Papillary maxillary labial frenum attached to the interdental papilla. **b,** A vertical incision is made along the center of the frenum from the gingival margin of the frenum to the vestibule. Two other incisions are then made, one at each end of the first incision. These two secondary incisions are made at approximately 60 degrees to the initial incision in opposite directions, forming a "Z". **c,** The mucosal flaps are then sutured in reverse position. This alters the fiber direction of the tissue from vertical to more horizontal and redistributes tension across the length of the incision. **d,** Healing provides a more apically relocated smaller frenum, an increased zone of attached gingiva, and reduced tension on the interproximal tissue.

Frenectomy

Frenectomy involves the complete removal of the frenum, including its attachment through periosteum to underlying bone.

      A. Simple frenectomy (Fig. 8-7).

      B. Classic frenectomy (Fig. 8-8).

      C. Frenectomy with vestibular sulcus extension (Fig. 8-9); Example includes orthodontic fiberotomy.

      D. Frenectomy with frenoplasty.

            1. lateral sliding flap

            2. free gingival graft

      E. Frenectomy by corticotomy.

Simple Frenectomy

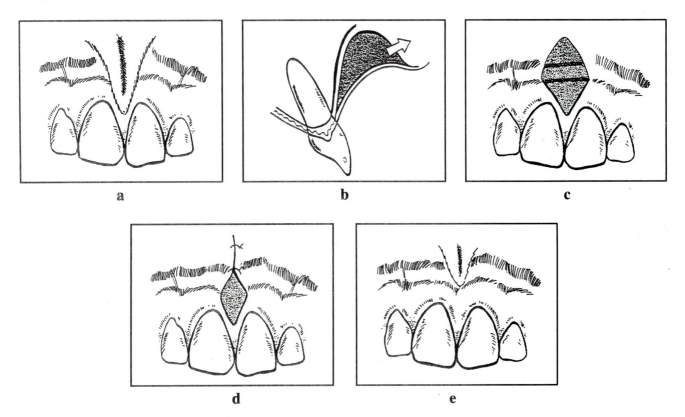

Fig. 8-7. a, Papillary attachment of maxillary labial frenum. **b**, Lateral view depicting extent of tissue to be excised (grey area). Lip is stretched outward and upward to judge the limits of the frenum and to provide surgical access. **c**, The frenum is excised with vertical incisions parallel to the borders of the frenum. The wound created is rhomboid in shape, with the widest part at the base of vestibule. The periosteum covering the labial plate of the alveolus thus exposed is fenestrated (scored) using a scalpel or curette. **d**, Mucosal tissues are sutured together to reduce wound area. Remaining exposed area will heal by secondary intention. **e**, Healing results in apically relocated, smaller frenum and increased zone of attached gingiva interproximally. Had this frenum penetrated through to the incisal papilla, a single vertical incision would be made through the center of the interproximal tissue to bone (orthodontic fiberotomy). This severs the interdental transseptal fibers.

Classic Frenectomy

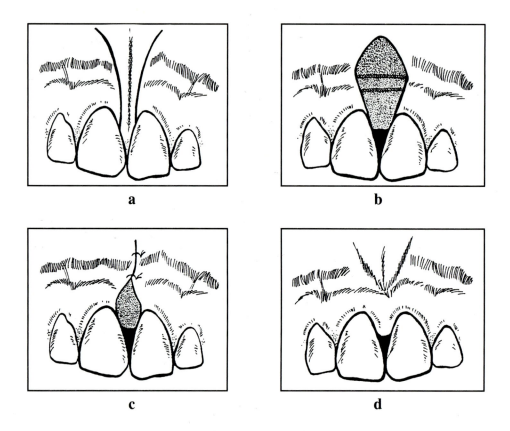

Fig. 8-8. **a**, Papillary penetrating frenum attaching to interproximal papilla and progressing between the teeth to the incisive papilla. **b**, Frenum is excised down to periosteum with incisions parallel to the lateral borders of the frenum. Periosteum is scored. Frenum tissue in the tip of the papilla is removed, extending palatal to the incisal papilla. **c**, Mucosal borders are appositioned and sutured. Any exposed periosteum is allowed to heal by secondary intention. **d**, After healing, the case exhibits an apically relocated and reduced frenum and an increased zone of attached tissue with no tension in the soft tissue border. Because of the removal of the interproximal tissue, however, tissue contours and esthetics are not ideal. For these reasons, this frenectomy method is not highly recommended.

Frenectomy with vestibular sulcus extension and orthodontic midline fiberotomy:

Indicated for a very broad frenum or multiple frenae or where increased vestibular depth is desired. The fiberotomy should be done whenever fibers extend to the incisive papilla.

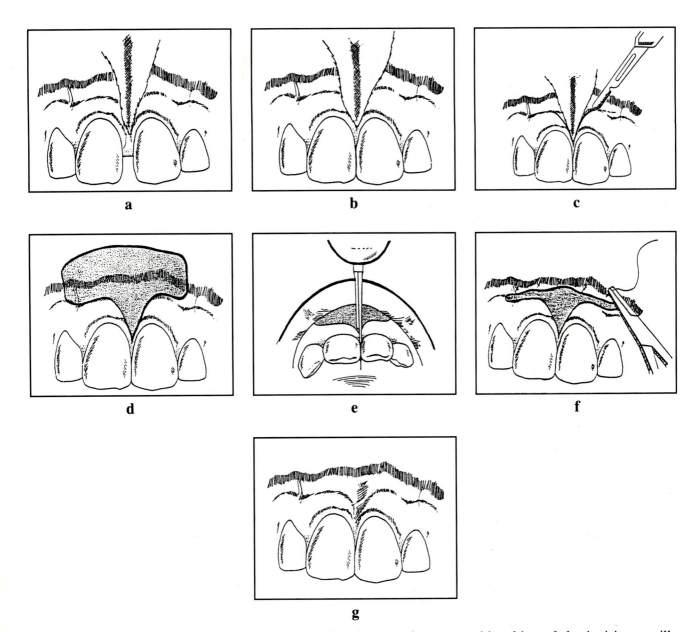

Fig. 8-9. **a,** Illustration of a papillary penetrating frenum that causes blanching of the incisive papilla when the lip is pulled (so-called "abnormal" frenum). This represents a patient over thirteen years of age and exemplifies that small percentage of the population (6-7%) in whom the diastema remains open even after the eruption of maxillary canines. **b,** After orthodontic closure. Retention is maintained with a maxillary retainer. **c,** This procedure begins with incisions that depart from the traditional V-shape by extending laterally one tooth's width along the mucogingival line. **d,** Tissue is reflected by sharp dissection, exposing thin bleeding connective tissue (periosteum). Bone is not necessarily exposed. Redundant tissue is excised. **e,** In order to sever elastic fibers between the central incisors, a scalpel is used to make an interproximal cut from the newly created wound palatally to the incisive papilla. No tissue is excised. However, the scalpel scrapes bone over a narrow area to insure complete separation of elastic fibers, allowing regrowth of connective tissue to teeth in the new closed relationship. **f,** The lip side of the wound is sutured to the periosteum, leaving a significant portion of the defect to heal by secondary intention. After healing, it will consist of attached gingiva. A horizontal fenestration in exposed periosteum is optional, depending on what the operator feels is the tendency for relapse. The use of a periodontal pack depends on operator preference. **g,** Final healing.

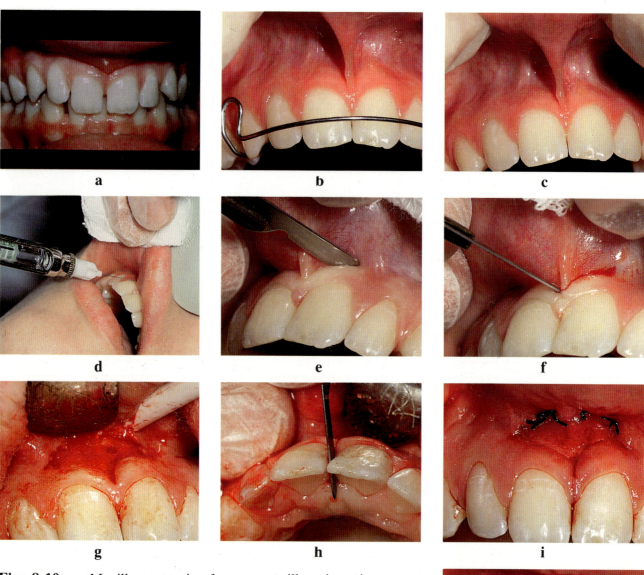

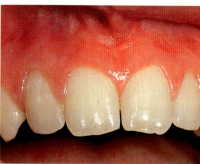

Fig. 8-10. a, Maxillary anterior frenum, papillary insertion—pre-orthodontic record. **b**, Postorthodontics—case in retention. **c**, Tension can be transmitted through the frenum to interdental tissues when the lip is stretched. **d**, Local anesthetic is administered using xylocaine 2% with 1:50,000 epinephrine. **e**, Initial incision. The surgical procedure follows the method outlined in Fig. 8-9. **f**, Continuation of the initial incision across the midline along the mucogingival line. **g**, Apical repositioning of the frenum and associated tissue with a partial-thickness reflection. Periosteum is exposed. **h**, Interproximal cut to sever elastic connective tissue fibers (see Fig. 8-9e). **i**, The cut edge of the mucosa is sutured to periosteum. To avoid relapse, it is advisable to place a barrier directly on the periosteum. For example, in this case a small piece of cloth (amalgam squeeze cloth) was cut to the dimensions of the wound, impregnated with FDA-approved cyanoacrylate, and placed quickly over the defect. It was left in position for one week. **j**, Postoperative healing.

Frenectomy with Frenoplasty

This type is indicated when a predictable increase in the zone of attached gingiva is needed.

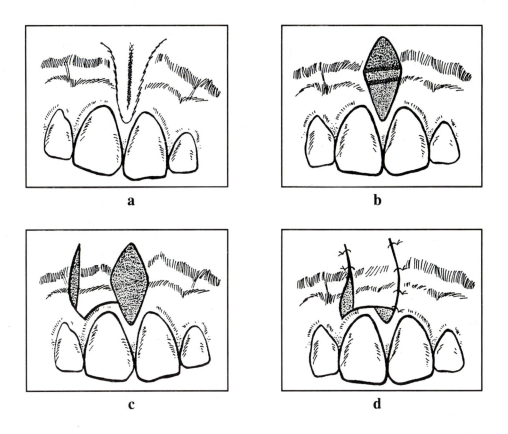

Fig. 8-11. Frenectomy with lateral sliding flap. **a,** Frenum attachment in the interproximal papilla. **b,** Basic excision of the frenum down to periosteum. Scoring of the periosteum is desirable, but do not remove periosteum. **c,** Pedicle flap of attached gingiva and mucosa is sharply dissected (split-thickness) from an adjacent site. Marginal gingiva is left intact to reduce the possibility of inducing marginal recession. **d,** A pedicle flap is moved medially and sutured into position over the wound area. The exposed area will heal by secondary intention. The healed result will prevent reattachment of the frenum and provide a predictable zone of attached gingiva. This procedure is more technique-sensitive than others and there is a risk of gingival recession over the donor tooth.

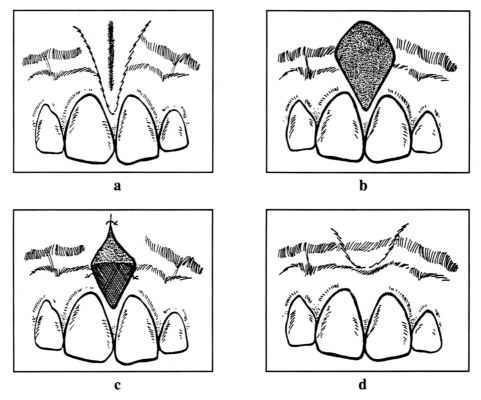

Figure 8-12. Frenectomy with free gingival graft. a, Papillary attachment of the maxillary labial frenum. **b**, Basic excision of the frenum down to the periosteum. Periosteum may be scored apical to the mucogingival line. **c**, Free gingival graft obtained from suitable donor site is sized and sutured in place. **d**, Healed result will provide an enhanced zone of attached gingiva with the frenum removed and prevented from reattachment.

Frenectomy by Osteotomy

Just as an abnormal frenum (one that exerts traction on the incisive papilla when the upper lip is stretched) is felt to contribute to the relapse of midline diastema closure if not surgically corrected, some clinicians also blame a patent intermaxillary bony suture for this problem.

Among those who view this phenomenon as a causative factor in diastema recurrence, the midline osteotomy (ostectomy) is the procedure of choice.[3-4] Krout[5] has reported no relapse with 28 patients on whom this procedure was performed.

Indications for the procedure are (1) significant midline diastema, (2) an open intermaxillary suture, (3) erupted permanent canines, and (4) desired permanent orthodontic closure of the midline space.

The technique consists of:

- Access by way of full-thickness flaps – facial and lingual.
- Osteotomy performed with a 701 fissure bur – obliterating the cortical lining of the intermaxillary suture. The cut includes both labial and palatal surfaces along with intervening bone and extends apically to the apices of teeth involved.
- Flap repositioning and suturing.
- Active orthodontic force. Rapid closure.
- Frenectomy is not necessary.

MANDIBULAR LABIAL FRENUM
Diagnosis and Treatment

Fig. 8-13, a and **b.** Labial and buccal frenae in the mandibular arch can present problems similar to those mentioned above with the maxillary arch. Although midline diastema problems are usually not a concern here, mandibular frenae are frequently associated with periodontal problems, such as inadequate or absent attached gingiva, mucogingival pockets, detachment of gingiva from root surfaces, and recession of the gingival margin.

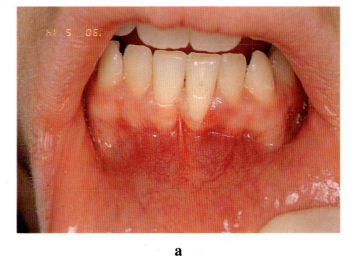

a

Surgical techniques such as those described for the maxillary labial frenum can be applied. Because of the different nature of the periodontium in this area (narrower zones of attached gingiva, thin labial attached gingiva, and shallow vestibular depth) successful treatment of the labial and buccal frenae in the mandibular arch generally requires apical relocation of the frenum, establishment of an enhanced zone of attached gingiva, and frequently coverage of denuded root surfaces as well. These objectives are best accomplished using frenectomy procedures combined with gingival grafting techniques as described in Chapter Two.

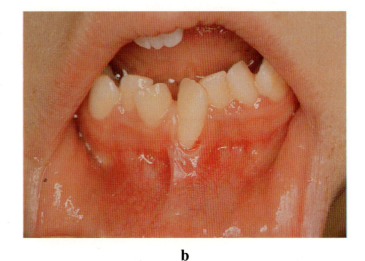

b

Fig. 8-14, a, This case exemplifies a clinical situation occasionally observed in the mouth. Labial to teeth numbers 24 and 25, we see the absence of attached gingiva, muscle pull on the free margin, and root exposure.

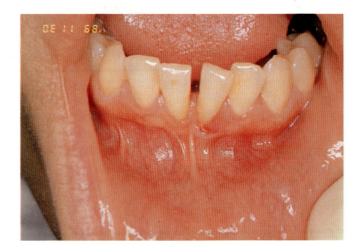

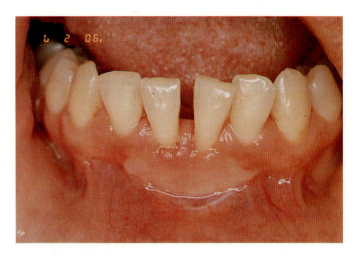

Fig. 8-14, b, A frenectomy alone would be inadequate in this instance. A successful free gingival graft, on the other hand, should satisfy requirements for more healthy periodontium.

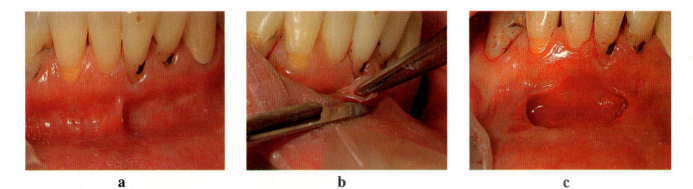

a   b   c

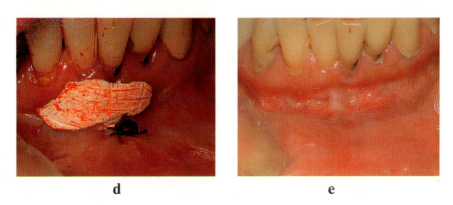

d   e

Fig. 8-15. a, The patient shown here was treated with frenectomy alone. The outcome was moderately successful. The muscle pull was alleviated, but the labial periodontium is still compromised. If the patient is to be subjected to a surgical procedure, it is usually better to broaden surgical objectives to include augmentation of attached gingiva and possibly even root coverage—both with a free autograft. **b**, Tissue excision. **c**, Exposure of periosteum. **d**, Pack placement over a wound that has been partially closed. Exposed periosteum is left to epithelialize secondarily. **e**, Postoperative healing.

TONGUE-TIE RELEASE IN CHILDREN

In infants, the lingual frenum is often attached near the tip of the tongue. This position usually changes with age, resulting in a more posterior connection. If by age four to seven, a child still has a short frenum with attachment close to the tip of the tongue and/or high on the alveolar process, surgical correction may be indicated to prevent possible speech abnormalities, lingual gingival defects, and dental malpositioning. A speech therapist should be consulted when surgical therapy is anticipated.[6]

When the tongue is tied flat in the floor of the mouth, it can place abnormal pressure against the lower incisors during speech and swallowing. This frequently causes labial tipping of the lower incisors. In addition, when the tongue is in this position, development of the palatal vault and maxillary arch may be more narrow than normal, leading to additional orthodontic problems including posterior crossbite.[6-7] If corrective surgery is performed early enough in the child's development and proper tongue habits are achieved, tooth position and arch form problems may be self-correcting.

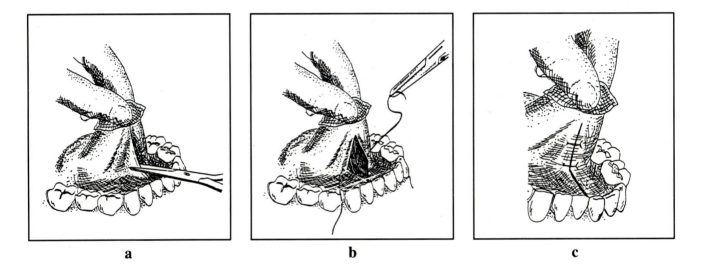

a   b   c

Fig. 8-16. Tongue-tie release by transverse incision. a, Anesthesia for this procedure may be local or general. If local anesthetic is used, bilateral lingual nerve blocks or local infiltrations can be used. Control of the tongue is essential for this procedure. This may be accomplished by grasping the tip of the tongue with a piece of gauze or with a traction suture placed through the tip of the tongue about 1/4 inch from the tip. The tongue is retracted forward and upward. Identify the opening of Wharton's ducts from the submandibular glands. Make a horizontal cut with surgical scissors or scalpel midway between the ventral surface of the tongue and the duct caruncles (about 1 cm above the duct openings). The incision extends to the muscle fibers of the tongue. After the initial incision, if there is still insufficient mobility of the wound margins for approximation when suturing, the margins can be undermined by inserting and opening the beaks of surgical scissors under the mucosal tissue. **b,** The diamond-shaped wound is sutured as a linear incision. On the ventral surface of the tongue the incision should be tightly closed. **c,** On the floor of the mouth, complete closure is not necessary and some clinicians place no sutures here at all. Avoid constriction of the salivary ducts by placing only superficial sutures through this mucosa.

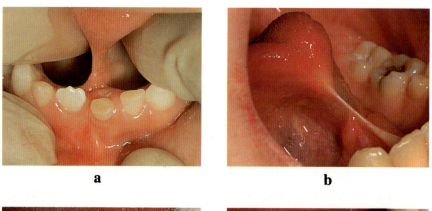

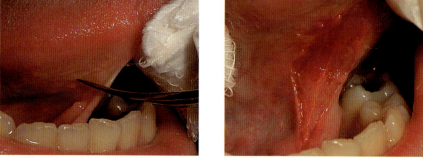

Fig. 8-17. a, This is an example of lingual tongue-tie. **b,** Another tongue-tie case. The patient was unable to articulate several speech sounds correctly. This may or may not be related to the anomalous anatomy. **c,** The tongue grasped with a piece of 2x2 gauze, following which the operator prepared to make a single transverse cut with surgical scissors. **d,** After this single cut is made, there is a characteristic vertical, diamond-shaped defect. **e,** First suture being placed. **f,** Suturing completed.

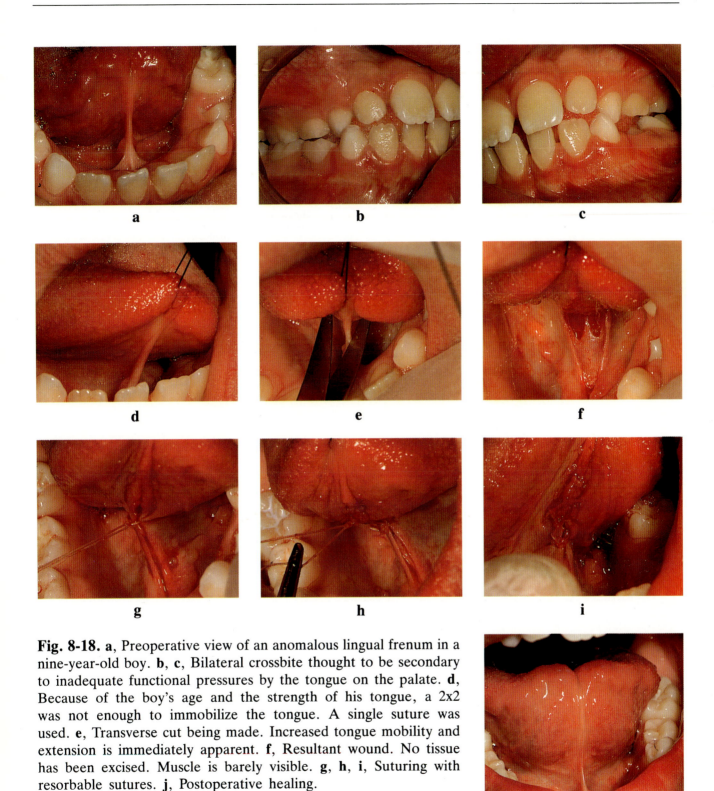

Fig. 8-18. a, Preoperative view of an anomalous lingual frenum in a nine-year-old boy. **b, c,** Bilateral crossbite thought to be secondary to inadequate functional pressures by the tongue on the palate. **d,** Because of the boy's age and the strength of his tongue, a 2x2 was not enough to immobilize the tongue. A single suture was used. **e,** Transverse cut being made. Increased tongue mobility and extension is immediately apparent. **f,** Resultant wound. No tissue has been excised. Muscle is barely visible. **g, h, i,** Suturing with resorbable sutures. **j,** Postoperative healing.

Table 8-3. Tongue-tie Release Flowchart

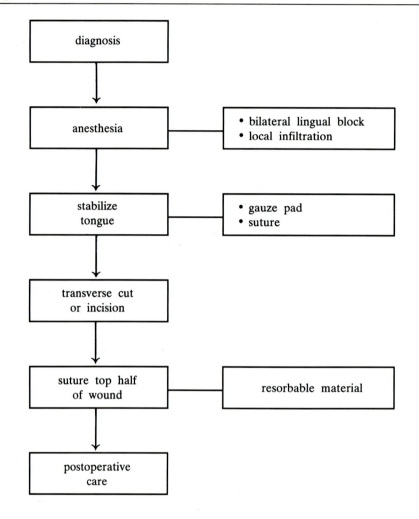

EDENTULOUS ARCH FRENAE

The maxillary labial frenum may become hypertrophied or develop insertions close to the crest of the alveolar ridge from extensive bone resorption. This then may result in an unesthetic appearance and can also affect denture retention through disruption of an adequate seal.

Surgical correction, if needed, is best done at the time of tooth extractions, but may be accomplished at a later date should it become necessary. A temporary reline material is added to the denture at the time of surgery to maintain soft tissue correction during healing, and a permanent reline or new prosthesis is constructed after complete healing.

The type of frenectomy procedure utilized frequently depends on the shape of the frenum. If it is thin and clearly defined, a simple surgical excision can be performed either by using V-shaped incisions (Fig. 8-20) or the double hemostat method. If the frenum is broad or has multiple attachments in the mucobuccal fold, it is better treated with a localized vestibuloplasty. Either method may be used as needed for any maxillary or mandibular frenum location.

Narrow Frenum Excision

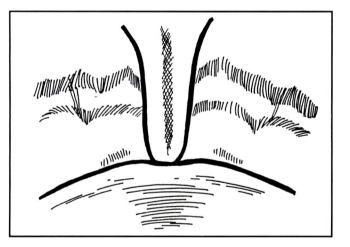

Fig. 8-19, a. Narrow frenum in edentulous arch. Inject the local anesthetic lateral to the surgical site to avoid distention of the tissues. Extend and evert the lip for access. V-shaped incisions are made through the mucosa lateral to the frenum. These incisions should extend from the frenum insertion on the lip to the attachment at the alveolar crest.

Fig. 8-19, b. Separate the frenum from adjacent tissues. In some cases this will be to the anterior nasal spine. Excise the frenum from soft tissue and bony attachment by sharp dissection with scissors or scalpel. Tissue tags and muscle fiber attachments thus exposed are trimmed away. Adjacent mucosa can be undermined by blunt dissection for approximately 2 cm laterally to facilitate wound closure.

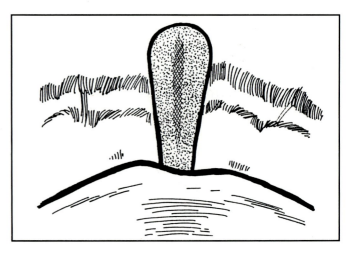

Fig. 8-19, c. To prevent frenum relapse, place the most apical suture (at the base of the vestibule) not only through the mucosal edges, but also securely through the periosteum. This effectively tacks the tissue down at the most apical position. Other interrupted sutures are placed as needed. Generally the wound cannot be completely approximated and a small area will heal by secondary intention.

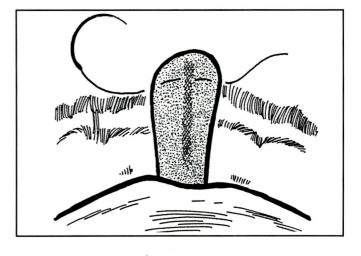

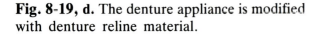

Fig. 8-19, d. The denture appliance is modified with denture reline material.

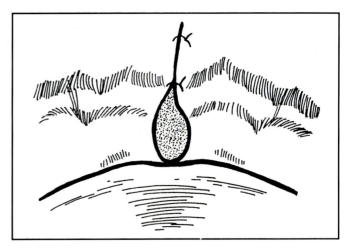

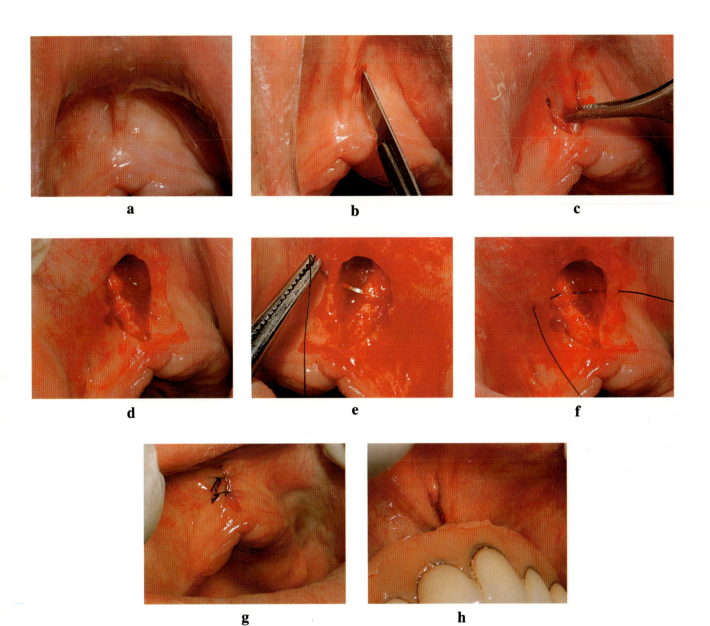

Fig. 8-20. a, This case exhibits an edentulous maxillary arch with a narrow anterior frenum that is very prominent, extending to the crest of the ridge. It interferes with the stability and retention of the maxillary denture. **b,** Initial incisions parallel the frenum on either side and extend to the mucobuccal fold. The scalpel can penetrate to bone. **c,** After the vertical incision lines are made, the frenum tissue is lifted with tissue pickups as the frenum is dissected underneath using a scalpel. **d,** Frenum tissue is removed completely down to the periosteum. **e,** The wound is sutured with the first suture passing through periosteum at the vestibular level. This suture is termed the "anchor" suture. **f,** The suture needle passes through the mucosa, periosteum, and the mucosa again. **g,** With very few sutures, the frenectomy wound can be closed with primary closure. Occasionally, a little lateral undermining is desirable to aid with closure. If some periosteum is not covered, it will heal uneventfully by secondary intention. **h,** The denture should be relined with a soft liner to help establish the new denture border.

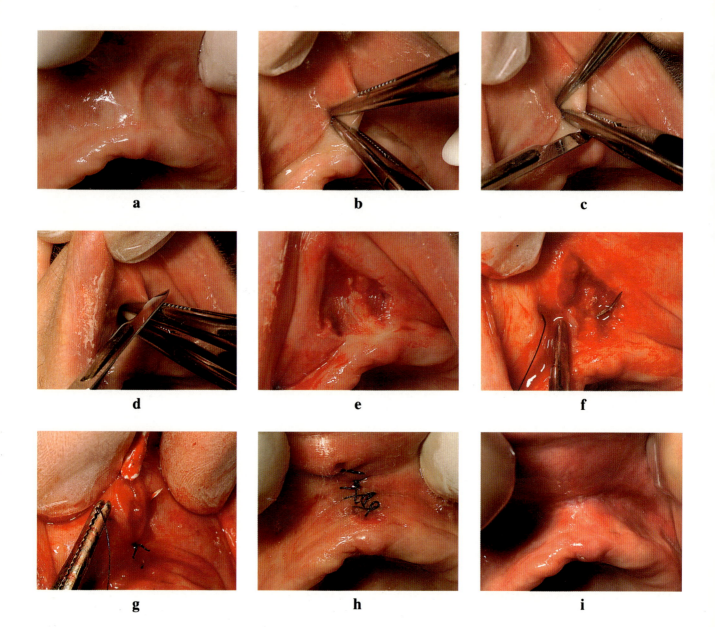

a

b

c

d

e

f

g

h

i

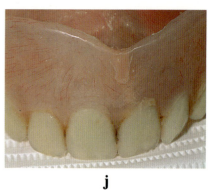

j

Fig. 8-21. a, Narrow frenum associated with an edentulous maxillary arch. The frenum extends to near the ridge crest. **b,** Two hemostats placed to guide the excision of unwanted tissue. One is positioned next to the alveolar ridge and the other is adjacent to the lip. **c, d,** A scalpel is used to cut along the outside surfaces of the hemostats, with the incisions meeting near the hemostat tips. **e,** Resultant wound. **f,** After minimal lateral undermining with the scalpel, the defect can be closed, beginning with the anchor suture. This suture passes through both mucosa and periosteum. **g,** Additional sutures are placed as needed. **h,** Closed wound. **i,** The denture is relined to the new vestibular depth to aid in maintenance of this extension. **j,** One week postop. A minimal adjustment of the flange is necessary to alleviate discomfort.

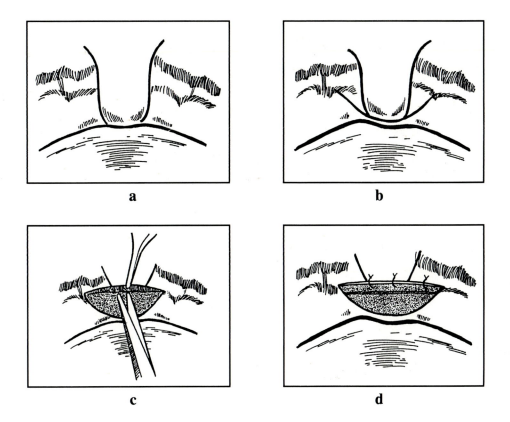

Fig. 8-22. Frenum excision for broad-based or multiple frenae. Recommended technique: Localized vestibuloplasty with secondary epithelialization.[6,8] **a,** Wide, broad-based frenum attaching to the edentulous ridge crest. Inject local anesthetic lateral to the surgical site to minimize tissue distension. Extend and evert the lip for access. **b,** Begin the localized vestibuloplasty by making a semilunar incision that exceeds the horizontal and vertical limits of the frenum. **c,** With scissors or scalpel, dissect and disengage the frenum from periosteum. Attached muscle fibers should also be cut during this process. As the dissection proceeds, retract the frenum/mucosal flap with tissue pickups. **d,** The frenum is excised at its apical border. The apical or mobile wound margin is sutured down to the periosteum at the level of the mucobuccal fold. The outer surface of the periosteum is left to re-epithelialize by secondary intention. The periosteum may be scored along the base of the newly created vestibule to further inhibit elastic fiber reattachment. The denture flange in this area is relined to the new vestibular contour.

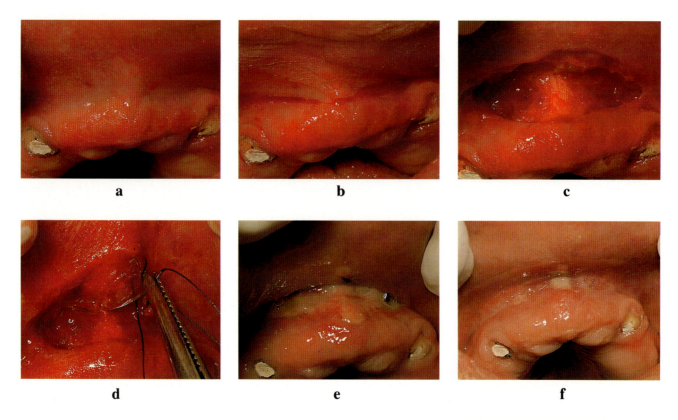

a

b

c

d

e

f

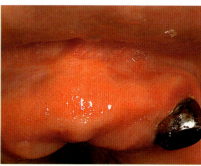

g

Fig. 8-23. a, This maxillary overdenture case has a broad anterior frenum that inserts almost at the crest of the edentulous ridge. It leaves a very limited vestibular depth in this area. **b,** The initial incision was a wide semilunar. **c,** A split-thickness flap was gradually apically repositioned, exposing about 1.5 cm vertical width of periosteal surface area. **d,** The mucosal border was sutured to the periosteum at the new vestibular level. **e,** The periosteum was scored (fenestrated) through to bone with a scalpel to discourage relapse of the frenum and to encourage replacement by attached tissue that is tightly bound to bone. **f,** Healing at five days. This wound is healing by secondary intention. **g,** Final healing. There is greatly increased vestibular depth, and the frenum now does not interfere with retention of the final prosthesis.

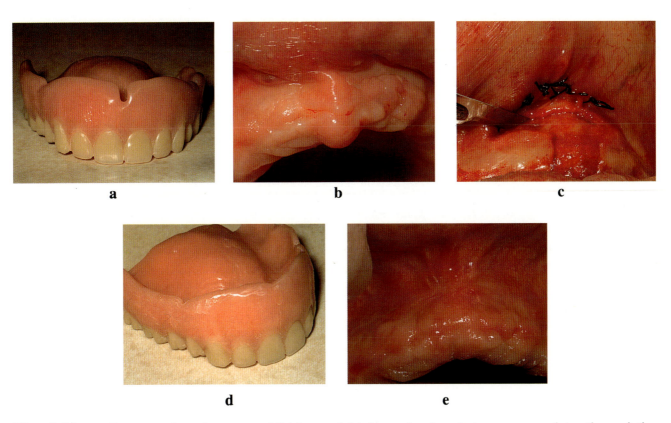

Fig. 8-24. a, Preoperative denture exhibiting a labial notch placed to accommodate the existing frenum. **b**, Preoperative clinical view. **c**, An exophytic nodule was excised from the ridge crest and the frenum repositioned apically, leaving periosteum exposed. This procedure could be termed a minor vestibuloplasty. A horizontal fenestration to bone was made along the apical aspect of the wound. **d**, The notch in the denture was filled in with temporary hard chairside reline material to help prevent relapse. **e**, Final healing.

References

1. Edwards JG. The diastema, the frenum, the frenectomy: a clinical study. *Am J Ortho*. 1977;71(5):489.

2. Placek M, Skach M, and Mrklas L. Significance of the labial frenum attachment in periodontal disease in man. Part 1, classification and epidemiology of the labial frenum attachment. *J Perio*. 1974;45:891.

3. Clark D. Immediate closure of labial diastema by frenectomy and maxillary ostectomy. *J Oral Surg*. 1968;26(4):273.

4. Spilka DJ, and Mathews PH. Surgical closure of diastema of central incisors. *Am J Orthod*. 1979;76(4):443.

5. Kraut RA, and Payne J. Osteotomy of intermaxillary suture for closure of median diastema. *JADA*. 1983;107:760.

6. Laskin DM. *Oral and Maxillofacial Surgery, Vol. 2*. St. Louis, Mo: CV Mosby Co; 1985.

7. Jones, PG. *Clinical Paediatric Surgery, Diagnosis and Management, ed. 2*. Oxford, Engl: Blackwell Scientific Publications Ltd; 1976.

8. Birn H, and Winther JE. *Manual of Minor Oral Surgery—A Step by Step Atlas*. Philadelphia, Pa: WB Saunders Co; 1982.

Additional Reading Material

1. Archer WH. *Oral and Maxillofacial Surgery*, 5th ed. Philadelphia, Pa: WB Saunders Co; 1975.

2. Cohen ES. *Atlas of Periodontal Surgery*. Philadelphia, Pa: Lea & Febiger; 1988.

3. Costich ER, and Waite RP. *Fundamentals of Oral Surgery*. Philadelphia, Pa: WB Saunders Co; 1971.

4. Grant DA, Stern IB, and Listgarten MA. *Periodontics*. St. Louis, Mo: The CV Mosby Co; 1988.

5. Hopkins R. *Color Atlas of Preprosthetic Surgery*. Philadelphia, Pa: Lea & Febiger; 1987.

6. Kinoshita S. *A Color Atlas of Periodontics*. St. Louis, Mo: Ishiyaku EuroAmerica; 1985.

7. Kruger E, and Worthington P. *Oral Surgery in Dental Practice*. Chicago, Il: Quintessence Publishing Co Inc; 1981.

8. Popovich F, Thompson GW, and Main PA. Persisting maxillary diastema: differential diagnosis and treatment. *J Canad Dent Assn*. 1977;7:330.

9. Sprigg RH. Double lingual frenotomy to correct the effects of retracted tongue position. Video tape produced by the Veterans Administration Dental Training Center.

10. Taylor JE. Clinical observations related to the normal and abnormal frenum labii superiorus. *Am J Ortho*. 1939;25:646.

11. Waite DE. *Textbook of Practical Oral Surgery*. Philadelphia, Pa: Lea & Febiger; 1978.

Chapter 9

Small Lesion Excision

INTRODUCTION

A clinical examination of the oral cavity will frequently reveal soft tissue lesions that require treatment. All dentists should be able to perform incisional or excisional biopsies, although in some cases the general dentist may feel that a referral to either an oral surgeon or physician is appropriate.

DIAGNOSTIC CRITERIA

Evaluation of a lesion usually includes a close visual inspection along with palpation of both the lesion and the surrounding area. Its history and all relevant findings should be recorded in detail in the patient's chart. A description should include the location, overall character, size, shape, surface texture, color, and the results of palpation. Regional lymph nodes should be examined. Any pulsation should be noted. Written descriptions and even sketches are helpful in monitoring possible changes in size or appearance. The patient's health history is important too, in that it may disclose information that could have a bearing on the final diagnosis. With this information at hand, a differential diagnosis can usually be made.

Lesions of traumatic origin will usually heal once the irritant is removed. However, follow-up visits should be scheduled regardless of the anticipated outcome. These types of lesions have been known to change into dangerous neoplasms.

After evaluating and following an oral soft tissue lesion for a reasonable length of time, the operator may feel that an incisional or excisional biopsy is necessary. Indications for biopsy and characteristics of malignant-looking lesions have been presented by Peterson[1] and are listed in Table 9-1.

Table 9-1. Indications for Soft Tissue Biopsy

1. A lesion that persists for over two weeks with no apparent etiologic basis.

2. A lesion that does not respond to treatment after 10-14 days, even after removing a local irritation.

3. Persistent hyperkeratotic changes in surface tissues.

4. A visible or palpable growth beneath relatively normal tissue.

5. Inflammatory changes of unknown cause that persist for long periods.

6. Lesions that interfere with local function, such as papillomas, fibromas, etc.

7. A lesion that has characteristics of malignancy. These could be:

- Erythroplasia - lesion is totally red or has a speckled red-and-white appearance.

- Ulceration - lesion is ulcerated or presents as an ulcer.

- Duration - lesion has persisted for more than two weeks.

- Rapid growth - lesion exhibits rapid growth.

- Bleeding - lesion bleeds on gentle manipulation.

- Induration - lesion and surrounding tissue is firm to the touch.

- Fixation - lesion feels attached to adjacent structures.

From Peterson LJ. *Contemporary Oral and Maxillofacial Surgery*. St. Louis, Mo.:CV Mosby Co.;1988.

As a rule, tumors suspected of malignancy should be referred to a surgical specialist. Generally, a confirmatory biopsy is best performed by the person who would treat the patient if follow-up surgery were necessary. An exception to this might be cases in which the dentist feels that the patient will not seek additional care, even when advised to do so, or when the practice is located in a remote area and valuable time may be saved by obtaining an immediate biopsy.[2] In these cases, the operator should, in most cases, go ahead with the excision.

General dentists may also want to defer to a specialist when the lesion is located in an area of anatomic uncertainty, such as the floor of the mouth, where an excision may be in close proximity to the ducts of major salivary glands, or in places where esthetics is a factor, such as near the vermillion border.

BIOPSY TECHNIQUES

Two common biopsy techniques are *incisional* and *excisional* biopsy. If the area under investigation measures over one centimeter, is in a location that would make excision difficult, or is suspected to be malignant, an incisional biopsy is indicated (see Fig. 9-1, a and b). This procedure removes only a representative piece of the lesion: such a sample should be wedge-shaped and include an adequate amount of normal as well as abnormal tissue. A deep, narrow sample is better than a broad, shallow one.

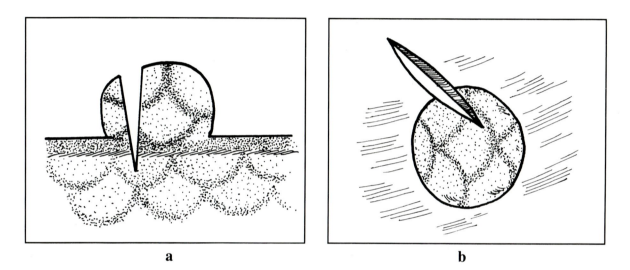

a	b

Fig. 9-1. Incisional biopsy, two views.

The excisional biopsy is used on small lesions that appear to be benign (see Fig. 9-2, a-h). These include: fibromas, lipomas, papillomas, small salivary adenomas, mucocoels, mucous cysts, gingival cysts, pyogenic granulomas and other similar lesions. It must be kept in mind that the defect created following excision will be about three times as large as the lesion itself since a set of elliptical incisions will be made, each clearing the lateral edges by 2-3 millimeters and joining at each end. The wide excision is meant to accomplish complete removal.

Pigmented and small vascular lesions should always be completely removed.[1] Not only does this removal constitute definitive treatment, in addition, the entire lesion is made available for histologic examination.

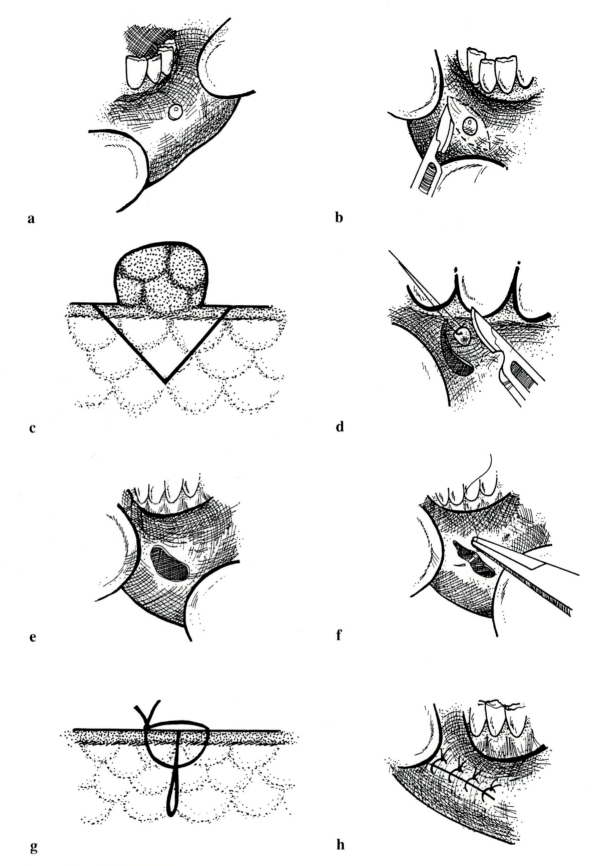

Figure 9-2. Excisional biopsy.

Table 9-2 gives suggestions for armamentarium to use during the procedure, and Figure 9-3 shows a tissue pickup, an instrument commonly used to provide traction on lesions during excision.

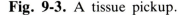

Table 9-2. Excisional biopsy armamentarium

1. Local anesthetic supplies
2. Scalpel with #15 blade
3. Tissue pickups
4. Gauze sponges
5. Needle holder
6. Suture material
7. Small hemostat
8. Surgical scissors
9. Biopsy report form

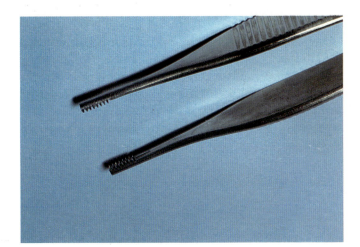

Fig. 9-3. A tissue pickup.

SURGICAL TREATMENT

Excisional Biopsy Technique

The step-by-step procedure for the excision of a small (under 1.0 cm) lesion is given below:

Step 1. Carefully evaluate the patient and the lesion, making full use of the health history, lesion history, and clinical examination results. Make a differential diagnosis. Decide who will perform the biopsy. Figure 9-4 gives an example of a lesion that should be removed.

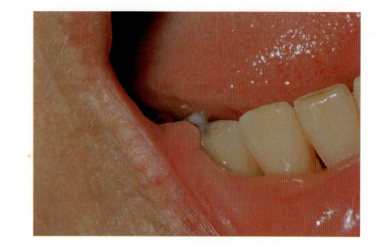

Fig. 9-4. Lesion that requires removal.

Step 2. Anesthetize the area with block anesthetic techniques if possible. When infiltration is used, it should be administered at least 1 cm away from the lesion (field block) to avoid artifactual distortion. Local anesthetic with 1:50,000 epinephrine helps provide hemostasis.

Step 3. Traction can be applied to the lesion by grasping the center with tissue pickups (*see Figure 9-5*). If it is felt that this may crush too much of the specimen, the lesion can be transfixed with one or more sutures, as shown in Figure 9-6. Sutures can be used to move and control the lesion and to tense the soft tissues during removal. Crushed tissue caused by pinching a large portion of the lesion with a hemostat may delay definitive diagnosis. Lips and similar tissue can be immobilized by tightening the tissue and stretching it with the thumb and index finger prior to removal (*see Figure 9-7*).

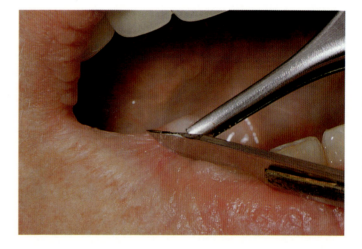

Fig. 9-5. Applying traction to lesion.

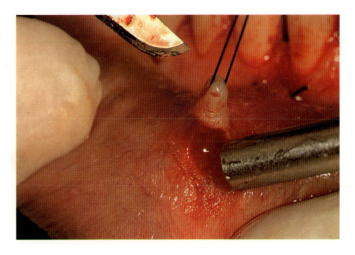

Fig. 9-6. Transfixing lesion with suture.

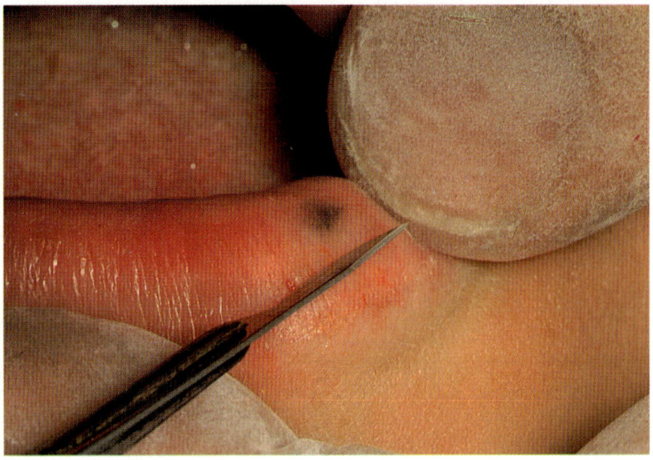

Fig. 9-7. Immobilizing tissue.

Step 4. With tension on the lesion, make elliptical incisions around it that join on the ends. These incisions should clear the lesion by 2-3 mm on either side and make V-shaped cuts that join under the specimen.[3] They should be planned to slightly exceed the depth of the specimen. To maintain tissue integrity, removal with a scalpel is preferable to electrosurgical excision.

The operator should try to make incisions parallel to the normal course of nerves and vasculature to prevent unnecessary trauma. In more vascular areas such as lips or the tongue, excessive bleeding may be controlled by having an assistant apply gauze under pressure (preferably soaked in warm water), and by picking up small bleeding points with curved "mosquito" hemostats. When the small hemostats are applied to bleeders for five minutes or so, it is rarely necessary to tie off the tissue, although this can be done if bleeding persists.

Step 5. After mucosa and underlying tissue have been incised, the lesion is separated from the surrounding area with a combination of sharp and blunt dissection. Figure 9-8 shows the defect resulting from complete excision.

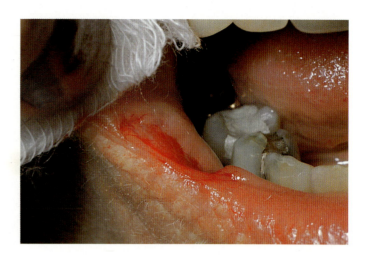

Fig. 9-8. Complete excision.

Step 6. The excised tissue is placed in a specimen jar with formalin, the appropriate paperwork (*see Table 9-4*) is completed, and the biopsy such as that shown in Figure 9-9 is sent to an oral pathology laboratory for a histologic examination.

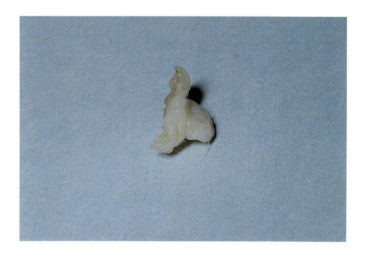

Fig. 9-9. Excised tissue.

Step 7. When the lesion is in unattached mucosa, as on the mucosal side of the lip or cheek, it may be desirable to undermine mucosal margins prior to suturing to facilitate primary closure.[4] This is done by placing the closed tips of pointed scissors into the submucosal area and spreading tissue by opening the scissor blades. In freely mobile tissue, undermining of the wound margins should be at least the width of the ellipse on all sides. This will allow easy approximation of the tissue with little or no tension on the sutures.

If the wound is in attached gingiva, it is often left to epithelialize by secondary intention. A pack may offer protection and increased comfort.

Step 8. The defect is usually closed with interrupted sutures. The first one is placed in the middle, and subsequent sutures are added on each side of the first to create more even closure (*see Figure 9-10*). Lesions under 1.25 cm generally do not require subcutaneous or muscle sutures. Sutures through mucosa should be 2-3 mm from the wound margin. Adjacent small mucous glands that are exposed can be excised with surgical scissor or scalpel. If they appear uninjured, they may be left in the wound.

In most cases, 3.0 or 4.0 silk suture material is appropriate. There are indications for other types in certain locations. Examples are (1) on the lips—where the operator may prefer 5.0 suture material, and (2) on the tongue—where resorbable material is usually advised because of discomfort during removal of silk.

Fig. 9-10. Placement of sutures.

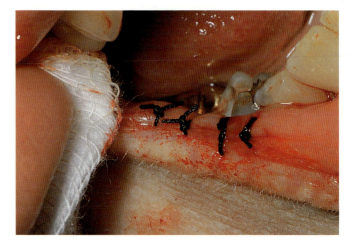

Step 9. Suture removal can be done five days postoperatively. The two-week postoperative examination usually demonstrates complete healing (Fig. 9-11). This lesion was diagnosed as an irritation fibroma. A summary of the treatment process is given in the flowchart in Table 9-3.

Fig. 9-11. Two weeks postoperatively.

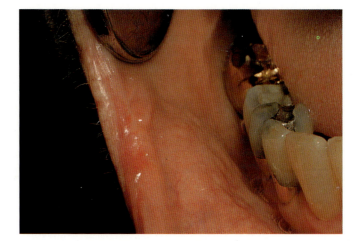

Step 10. The dentist should arrange a time to discuss the oral pathologist's findings with the patient after the laboratory results are returned (1-2 weeks). Oral pathologists should be utilized rather than general pathologists because of the former's familiarity with the rather unique nature of oral pathology.

Table 9-3. Contents of the Biopsy Report

The biopsy report form, which is usually provided with the specimen jar from the oral pathologist, should include the following information:

1. Date

2. Patient data:

> name
>
> address
>
> telephone number
>
> billing information (employer, insurance company, etc.)

3. Name, address, and telephone number of the doctor submitting the specimen

4. Other patient information, such as:

> gender
>
> occupation
>
> race
>
> age

5. Relevant findings from the patient's dental record or health history

6. Detailed history of the lesion

7. Presence of clinical signs or symptoms that could be related to the lesion, such as pain, edema, lymphadenopathy, and so on

8. Exact location of the lesion

9. Clinical appearance of the lesion:

> size
>
> color
>
> shape
>
> texture

10. Nature of treatment, i.e. excisional biopsy

Table 9-4. Small Lesion Excision Flowchart

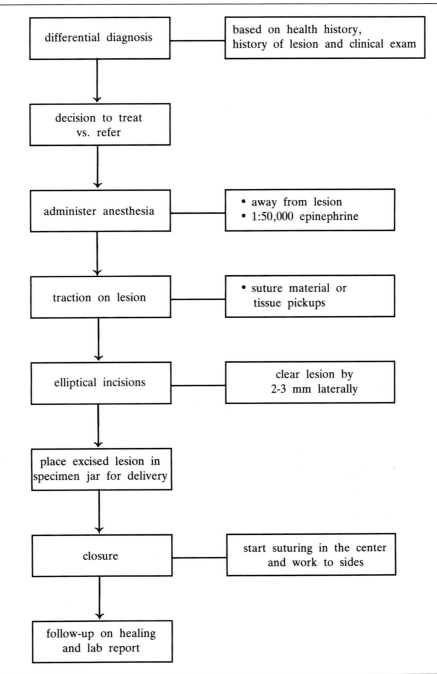

CLINICAL CASES

Case 1
Fibroma Excision

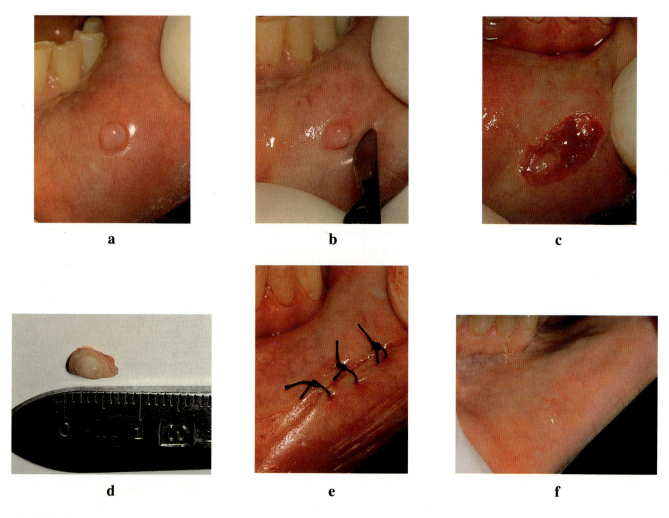

Fig. 9-12. a, A 62-year-old man presented with this lesion on the mucosal side of his lower lip. It was anesthetized by placing local anesthetic near the corner of his mouth and mucobuccal fold. This avoided distention of the area and distortion of the lesion from placing it too close. b, The operator is ready to begin the initial incision. Tissue pickups will be used to distend the lesion. c, Lesion excised. d, Specimen ready to place in formalin. e, Sutured lesion. f, Two-week postoperative appearance. The lab report confirmed an irritation fibroma.

Case 2
Fibroma Excision

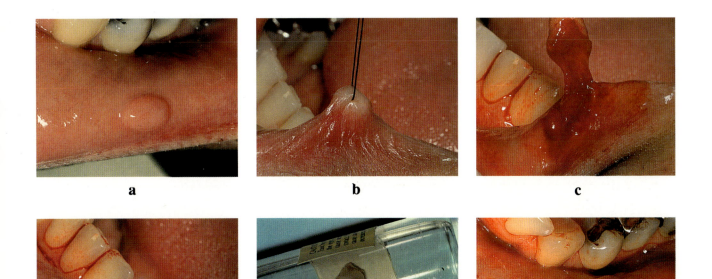

a

b

c

d

e

f

Fig. 9-13. a, A 45-year-old man presented with this lesion on the inside of the lower lip. **b**, Suture traction. **c**, Lesion in the process of excision. **d**, One suture placed. Note the mucous glands on the left side of the suture protruding from the wound. **e**, Specimen in jar of formalin ready to be sent to the lab. **f**, Sutured lesion. The lesion and resultant wound in this case was approximately twice as large as the previous two examples. **g**, Two-week postoperative appearance.

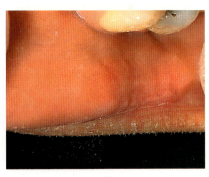

g

Case 3
Capillary Hemangioma Excision

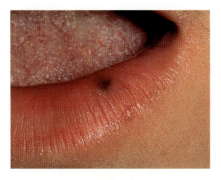

a

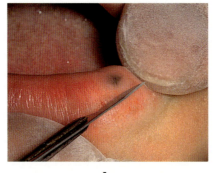

b

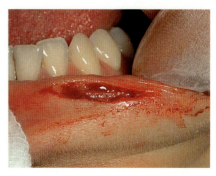

c

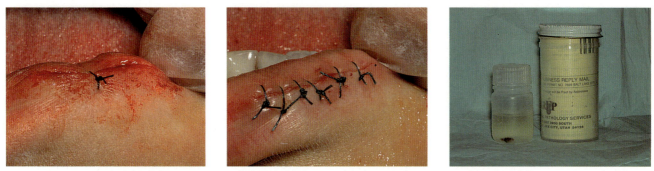

d

e

f

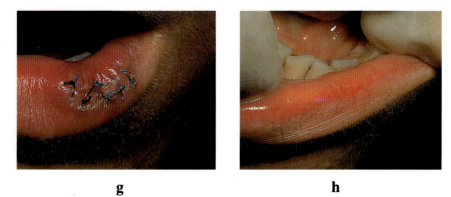

g

h

Fig. 9-14. a, A 21-year-old girl presented with this longstanding pigmented lesion on her lower lip that had remained unchanged for several years. **b**, Scalpel ready for incision. **c**, Lesion removed. **d**, One suture placed, bringing wound margins together at the center. **e**, Two additional sutures have now been added on either side of the first one, creating primary closure. **f**, Lesion ready to submit for histologic examination. **g**, Five-day postoperative appearance. **h**, Two-week postoperative appearance.

Case 2 Pathology Report

Gross Description:

The specimen consists of a raised, smooth, round, white soft tissue measuring 0.8 cm in diameter and up to 0.8 cm in depth. The tissue is bisected prior to processing.

Microscopic Description:

Sections reveal a portion of soft tissue covered by keratinized stratified squamous epithelium. In the central area the tissue is dome-shaped due to a large increase in the amount of randomly placed, interlacing, dense collagen bundles. In this area there are also vascular channels, fibroblasts and a few mononuclear inflammatory cells. At the deep margin of excision, nerve bundles, vascular channels and skeletal muscle are seen.

Diagnosis:

Irritation fibroma; lower left lip.

Case 3 Pathology Report

Gross Description:

Submitted in formalin is a soft tissue specimen measuring 1.6 x 0.8 x 0.9 cm in greatest dimensions. The specimen is bisected and submitted for processing.

Microscopic Description:

Microscopically the specimen is that of a capillary hemangioma characterized by an abundance of endothelial lined small spaces filled with red blood cells within a loose fibrous connective tissue. The specimen is surfaced by a stratified squamous cell epithelium.

There is no evidence of malignancy.

Diagnosis:

Capillary Hemangioma

Case 4
Irritation Fibroma Excision

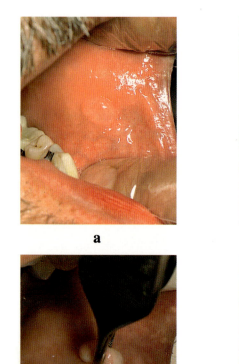
a

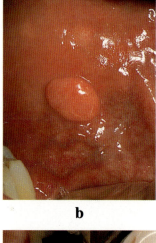
b

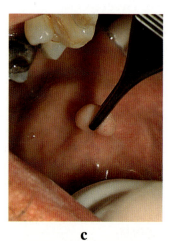
c

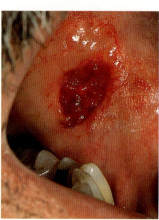
d

e

f

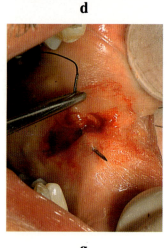
g

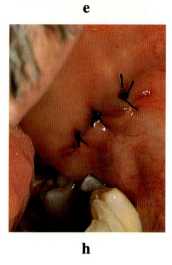
h

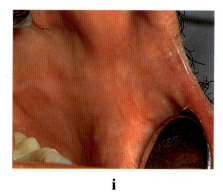
i

Fig. 9-15. **a**, General view of lesion on the inside of the cheek near the level of the occlusal plane. **b**, Close-up view. **c**, Traction on the lesion. **d**, The operator is ready to make the first incision. **e**, Lesion partially excised. **f**, Resultant surgical defect. **g**, First suture. **h**, Sutured wound. **i**, Two-week postoperative appearance. The lab report confirmed an irritation fibroma.

Case 5
Verruca Vulgaris Excision

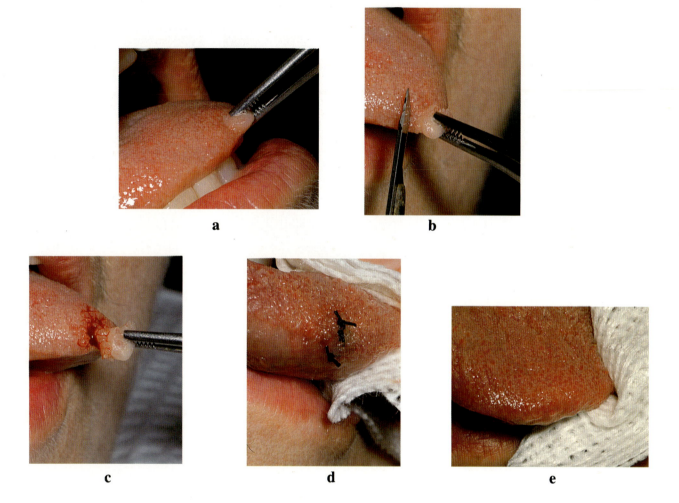

Fig. 9-16. a, Traction on the lesion. **b,** The operator is ready to make the first incision. **c,** First incision completed. **d,** Lesion closed with three silk sutures. Chromic gut could also have been used. The silk sutures were painful to remove. Chromic gut lasts about 9-14 days and would allow adequate healing prior to dissolving. Plain gut dissolves in 5-7 days and may give way too soon while the polyglycolic acid/polylactic acid-type materials remain for nearly one month and could be a nuisance to the patient following initial healing. **e,** Two-week postoperative appearance. The lab report confirmed a verruca vulgaris.

Case 6
Vascular Malformation Excision

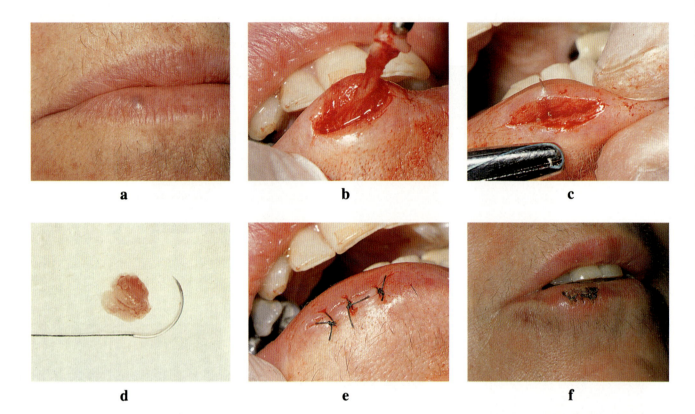

a   b   c

d   e   f

Fig. 9-17. a, Bluish lip lesion on a 55-year-old woman. She requested that it be removed because of its unesthetic appearance. **b**, The lesion was excised with elliptical incisions in a horizontal manner so as not to cross the vermillion border and to be in line with lip vasculature. **c**, The first suture is being placed. **d**, Lesion ready to submit for histologic examination. **e**, Sutured lesion. **f**, Five-day postop—sutures ready to be removed. **g**, Two-week postop view. On the pathology report, the lesion was listed to be a vascular malformation.

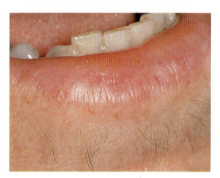

g

References

1. Peterson LJ. *Contemporary Oral and Maxillofacial Surgery*. St. Louis, Mo: CV Mosby Co; 1988; 473.

2. Kruger E, and Worthington P. *Oral Surgery in Dental Practice*. Chicago, Il: Quintessence Publishing Co Inc; 1981.

3. Birn H, and Winther JE. *Manual of Minor Oral Surgery – A Step by Step Atlas*. Philadelphia, Pa: WB Saunders Co; 1975.

4. Laskin DM. *Oral and Maxillofacial Surgery*. Vol. 2. St. Louis, Mo: CV Mosby Co; 1985.

Other Reading Materials

Howe GL. *Minor Oral Surgery*. 3rd ed. Bristol, England: John Wright and Sons Ltd; 1985.

Chapter 10

Removing Non-Impacted Teeth and Roots: From Routine to "Surgical"

INTRODUCTION

Nearly all general dentists are prepared to perform exodontia. Some practitioners feel uneasy engaging in these procedures because of the potential for unexpected complications. There is no guarantee that any tooth will be easily withdrawn from a socket. In fact, 10-20% of all extractions will inevitably require special means for their "surgical" removal. Even experienced dentists have teeth fracture in the process of removal. However, by using the established, step-by-step methods for difficult extractions presented in this chapter, most worry and guesswork can be eliminated.

After reviewing the instructions and case reports that follow, an operator will approach extractions more efficiently and will have the knowledge to anticipate and manage problems more competently should they occur.

Preparatory requirements for tooth removal include conducting the following:

1. A thorough patient assessment, including

   • health history

   • dental history

   • nature of the current dental problem

2. A clinical evaluation of the tooth and regional anatomy

3. A radiographic evaluation of the tooth and surrounding structures

4. Confirmation of indications for extraction

With these steps completed, dentist and staff can then commence with the actual surgery. There are three sections in this chapter dealing with instructions for tooth removal. They are:

Routine Removal,

More Difficult Cases, and

"Surgical" Extraction Procedures (involve flap reflection and bone removal).

The author acknowledges appreciation to the Ogram System™ of Exodontia for some of the concepts included in this chapter.

ROUTINE REMOVAL

Step 1. Reflect cervical gingiva to expose crestal bone. This protects marginal gingiva from being bruised or torn during the extraction process.

Step 2. Luxate the tooth or root in its socket. Luxation provides simultaneous bone expansion and periodontal ligament (PDL) disruption. Solid pressure should be exerted for 10 seconds or so, followed by a brief waiting period (a couple of minutes) to allow for increased hydrostatic pressure within the ligament space.[1] The sequence can be repeated if needed. This is done before elevation is attempted.

Use one or more of the following applications:

   A. *Wedge an elevator into the PDL* as close to the long axis of the tooth or root as possible, firmly engage the elevator, and then rotate with binding pressure against bone. After this luxating, forceps may be applied for additional luxation or removal. (See Fig. 10-1).

Fig. 10-1, a-c. Wedging an elevator into the PDL.

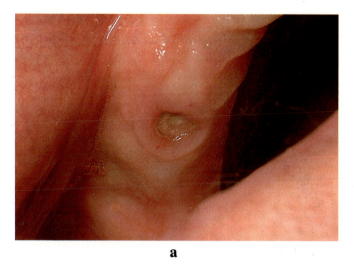

a

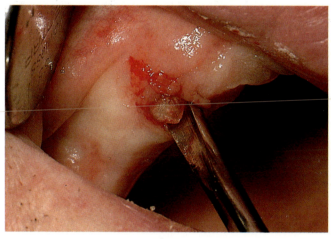

b

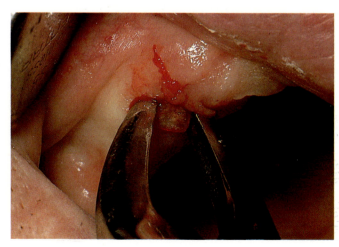

c

B. *Place a straight elevator* into the interdental space perpendicular to the tooth, use adjacent bone as a fulcrum, and rotate the superior sharp edge of the elevator against the tooth (Fig. 10-2a). Engaging the elevator in this manner serves to luxate the tooth. Rotating the lower, sharp edge of the elevator coronally into the cementoenamel junction both luxates and elevates (Fig. 10-2b). Application in both directions is described in dental literature. Do not involve the adjacent tooth unless it is also being extracted.

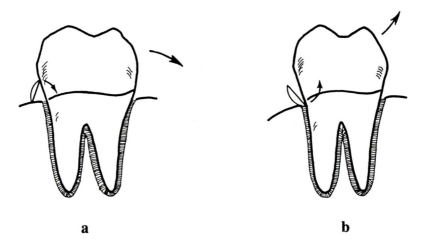

a   b

Fig. 10-2, a and b. Placing a straight elevator into the interdental space.

C. *Apply forceps pressure* (Fig. 10-3).

- facially and lingually (greater force facially except on lower molars)
- rotationally with firm reciprocation (See Figs. 10-1c and 10-3)

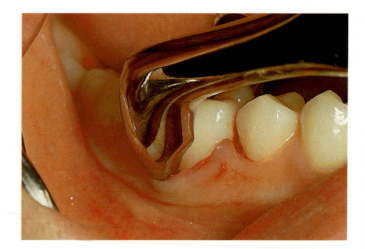

Fig. 10-3. Applying forceps pressure.

Step 3. Elevate the tooth or root out of its socket.

Apply one or more of the following:

> **A.** *Leverage of an elevator against the tooth using an adjacent fulcrum of bone.*
>
>> • Crane pick - generally used with a purchase point (Figs. 10-4 and 10-5)
>>
>> • straight elevator

Fig. 10-4.

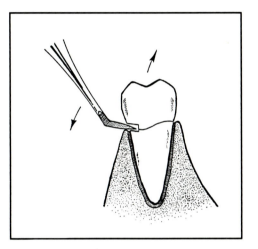

Fig. 10-5.

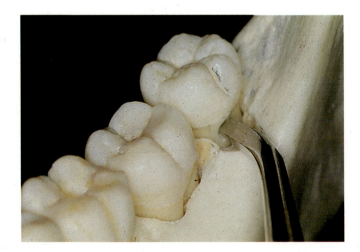

B. *Use of wheel and axle rotation.*

- pennant-shaped elevator (such as Cryer) to remove molar roots (Fig. 10-6)

  These elevators are effective only if applied at an angle less than 45 degrees. The large Cryer is used in the maxillary arch and the small one in the mandibular arch because of access limitations.[1]

- side of a straight elevator is rotated upward into the tooth (Fig. 10-2b)

Fig. 10-6.

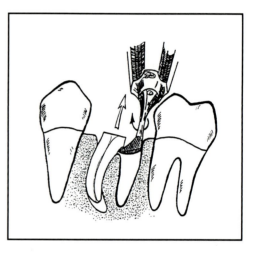

C. *Wedging of an elevator apically into the PDL space*—Causes bone expansion and tooth displacement (Figs. 10-7 through 10-9).

Fig. 10-7.

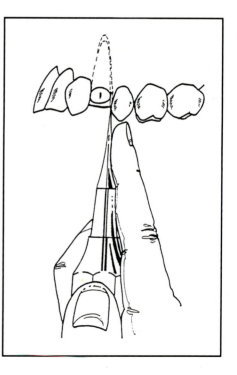

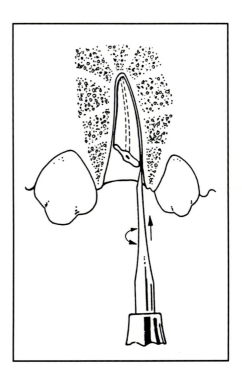

Fig. 10-8.

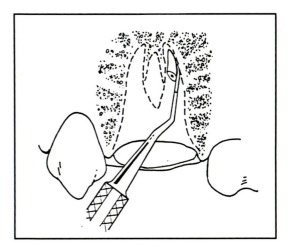

Fig. 10-9.

D. *Use of controlled traction with a forcep*—gentle pulling force to "walk" the tooth or root out of the socket (Fig. 10-10).

- tooth forcep
- root tip forcep

Fig. 10-10.

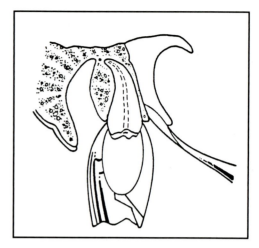

Step 4. Implementation of other, less conservative methods.

If, without using excessive force, the extraction attempt is unsuccessful because of reasons listed further in this writing, then other methods such as sectioning and bone removal will need to be used.

Table 10-1. Suggestions with Forcep Use

1. Forcep beaks should be applied in the long axis of the tooth to avoid root fracture.

2. The lingual beak of the forcep is usually seated first and then the buccal beak.

3. The operator should grasp handles of the forceps at their ends to maximize mechanical advantage and control.

4. The more apical the forcep beak placement, the lower the center of rotation and consequently, the lesser the probability of root fracture.

5. Use slow, steady facially and lingually directed forces with the forcep to expand the bone. These forces should generally be greater to the facial side (weaker bone) except with lower molars, where they often require stronger lingual forces (weaker bone on the lingual).

6. Forcep rotation on curved or multi-rooted teeth can predispose root fracture if excessive force is used.

7. Forcep traction forces are gentle and are reserved for the final stages of the extraction process.

8. The primary purpose of a forcep is not as much to quickly remove the tooth as it is to slowly expand the bone.

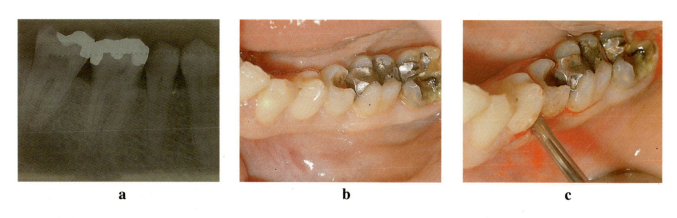

a   b   c

d   e   f

Fig. 10-11. a, This patient was adamant in his request for removal of this mandibular second premolar. **b**, Clinical view. **c**, Luxation was initially attempted with a 301 elevator. This was stopped because the elevator was also luxating the first premolar. **d**, Forcep luxation followed by forceps removal. **e**, Manual pressure to reposition bone following socket expansion on removal. **f**, Extracted tooth.

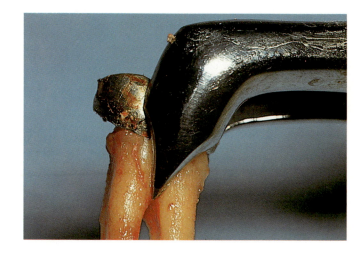

Fig. 10-12, a. Adaptation of the 79AS forcep on a recently extracted lower molar. Alternative forceps are the 17 or 23 (cowhorn).

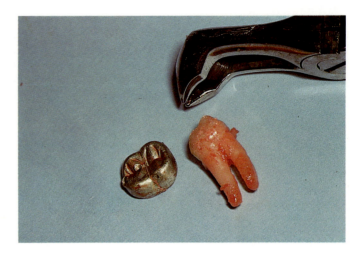

Fig. 10-12, b. Forcep and extracted tooth.

Table 10-2. Other Principles to Consider During Extraction.
(Adapted from Peterson, L.J., *Contemporary Oral and Maxillofacial Surgery*, The C.V. Mosby Company, 1988.)

1. Forceps are the major instrument for tooth luxation in most instances.

2. The straight elevator is inserted into the interdental space...perpendicular to the tooth. The inferior portion of the blade rests on the alveolar bone and the superior or occlusal portion of the blade is turned toward the tooth being extracted (Fig. 10-2a).

3. In certain situations, the elevator can be turned in the opposite direction (occlusal portion of the blade rotated up and away from the tooth being extracted) and more vertical displacement of the tooth will be achieved...

4. Surgeons should consider performing an elective surgical extraction anytime they perceive a possible need for excessive force to extract a tooth.

Table 10-3. Helpful Hints for Two Problem Situations

1. **For canine removal:** Lateral incisors and first premolars should be removed after canines to help avoid labial plate fracture. They offer needed support during the extraction of canines.

2. **For maxillary first premolar removal:** When removing maxillary first premolars, fracture of the palatal root can be minimized by avoiding strong forces to the palatal side. If a fracture does occur, it will most likely be the buccal root which is more accessible and further from the sinus. A buccal root tip can be teased out with a root tip pick (see Fig. 10-9) or via the flap/apical bony fenestration method (see Fig. 10-33).

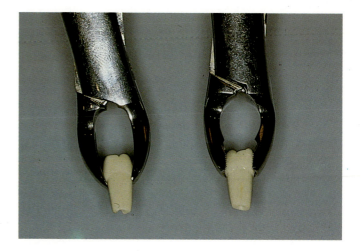

Fig. 10-13. Forcep design has a great impact on operator control of the tooth during removal. On the right, a conventional 150 upper universal forcep is shown grasping an ivorine premolar. Note the limited contact area of the instrument against the tooth. On the left, a different forcep (150AB) is holding a similar tooth, but exhibits about 10 times the contact area.

MORE DIFFICULT CASES

For teeth with multiple roots that do not come out easily because of divergence, curvatures, or when crowns are severely decayed or fractured, divide the root complex into single geometric components and remove them using the principles for "routine extractions" given previously. A few other helpful suggestions are also provided in this section. This process does not require extensive flap reflection or bone removal (*see Figs. 10-14 through 10-16*).

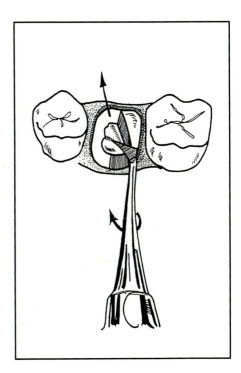

Fig. 10-14. Use of a small Cryer to remove a mandibular first molar mesial root following sectioning of the root complex and removal of the distal root.

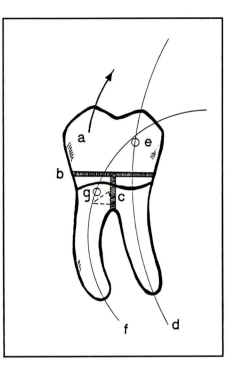

Fig. 10-15. Mechanics of Cryer usage.[1] **a**, Crown's path of removal. **b**, Horizontal section cut separating crown from roots. **c**, Vertical section cut separating the mesial and distal roots. **d**, Line corresponding to the distal root curvature. **e**, Apogee of the distal curved line. **f**, Line corresponding to the mesial root curvature. **g**, Apogee of the mesial curved line. The Cryer elevator must engage the root at or below the apogee at no greater than a 45-degree angle in order for the root to come out in a predictable manner.

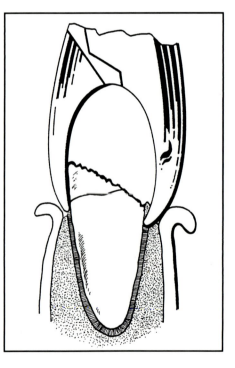

Fig. 10-16. Excision of bone with the buccal beak of a forcep during engagement of the tooth for extraction.

Fig. 10-17, a. As illustrated in Fig. 10-16, the buccal forcep beak here engages bone in an effort to remove a fractured root.

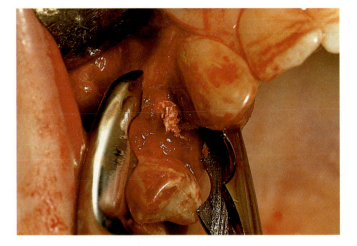

Fig. 10-17, b. Root and bone removed.

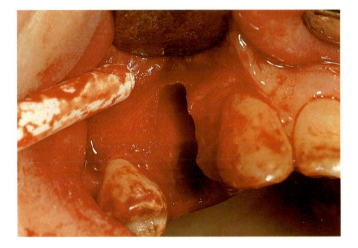

Fig. 10-17, c. Sutured case.

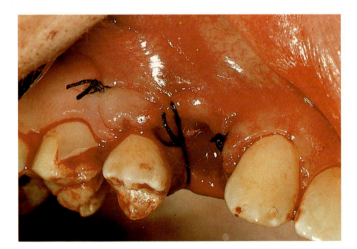

When multi-rooted teeth are being removed, one or more roots sometimes exhibit stubborn resistance. In these cases, a bur can be used to carefully excise bone located between the roots, using brush strokes and good irrigation (Fig. 10-18).

This accomplishes three things. First, it essentially eliminates about one fourth of the ligament attached to the root; second, it creates space for elevator instrumentation; and third, it provides a bare root surface into which the appropriate elevator (such as a Cryer) can be set. This is all done without enlarging the basic wound size and without endangering anatomic structures that may exist in hard tissue adjacent to the root area.

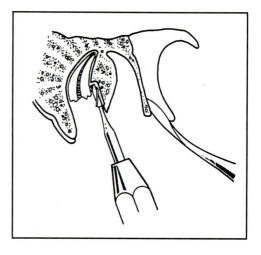

Fig. 10-18. Inter-radicular bone removal.

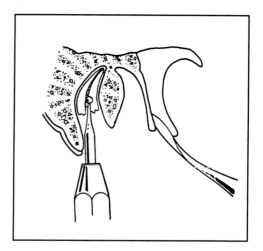

Fig. 10-19. Another way to complete extractions without the invasiveness of flap reflection and extensive bone removal is with a straight handpiece and #6 round bur. The bur is stalled in the root and then traction is applied using the handpiece (Fig. 10-19).

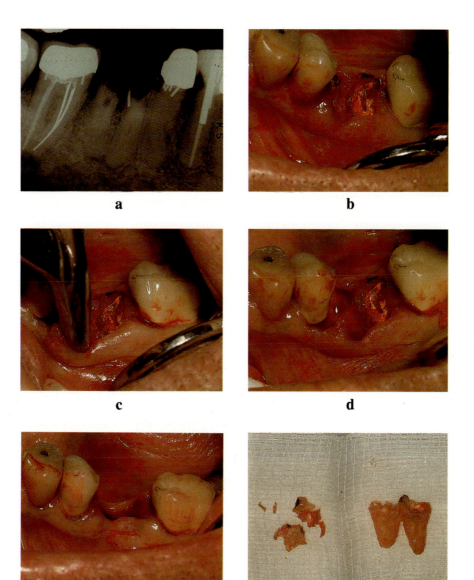

Fig. 10-20. a, A 65-year-old man presented with a fractured tooth. **b**, Clinical view. **c**, After reflection of cervical gingiva, the mesial root was engaged with a forcep. A section cut was not made with the bur because the x-ray indicated that the roots were already separate. **d**, The distal root was grasped in a similar manner. **e**, With both roots removed, the case was then sutured. **f**, Root fragments.

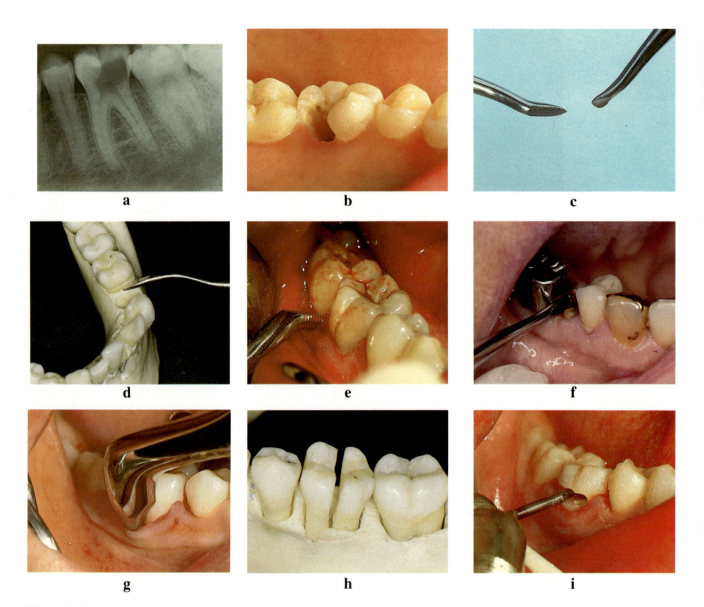

Fig. 10-21, a-i. This figure illustrates the removal of a lower first molar with nonrestorable caries. a, X-ray. b, Clinical view. c,Two instruments used with the Ogram System having the capability of luxating a single tooth without traumatizing the adjacent tooth. Left, 77R. Right, 98. d, The 77R is shown in position. Instead of rotating the instrument as with conventional straight elevators placed interproximally, the inferior serrated edge of this elevator is engaged against the tooth's cementoenamel junction (CEJ) while its handle is moved apically. e, This motion elevated the working end coronally, causing luxation and elevation of the tooth. Buccal interproximal bone serves as the fulcrum. The 98 functions according to the same principle, but allows the operator to (1) work in a more narrow interproximal space (only the tip of the instrument is used) or (2) where bone loss has increased the distance from crestal bone to the CEJ (this instrument is longer than the 77R). f, This conventional straight elevator may luxate the fractured root, but it will probably also loosen the adjacent crown in the process. g, Firm, but not heavy reciprocating and buccolingual forces are applied to luxate this tooth. This causes bone expansion and an increase in hydrostatic pressure within the periodontal ligament (PDL). h, This is one method used by practitioners to section a lower molar with divergent roots—especially if the crown is solid. The tooth may still fracture in half at the crestal bone level. i, Since this tooth has been severely weakened with decay, the tooth is being sectioned horizontally at the gingival margin prior to being sectioned between the roots.

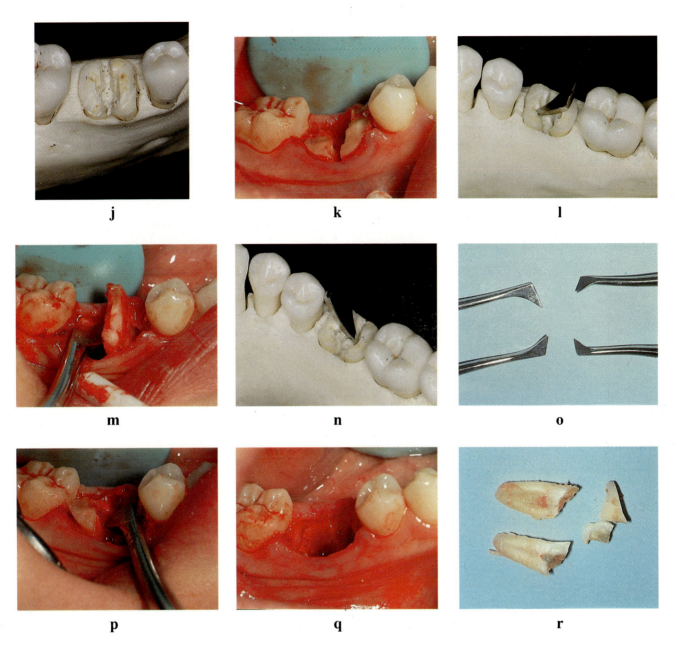

j   k   l

m   n   o

p   q   r

Fig. 10-21, j-r. j, Crown removed. **k**, A section cut was made with a 1702 bur followed by confirmation of separation with a straight elevator. **l**, The small Cryer uses the distal root as a fulcrum to luxate and elevate the mesial root. **m**, Root during elevation. **n**, This picture illustrates why the large Cryer is not used in the mandibular arch. Its application can cause serious damage to an adjacent tooth. **o**, Comparison in size between large and small Cryer elevators. **p**, Distal root being removed. **q**, Extraction completed. **r**, Tooth fragments.

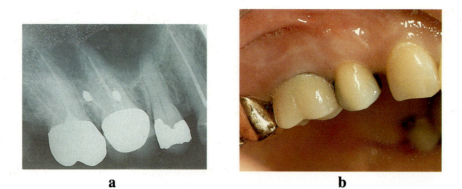

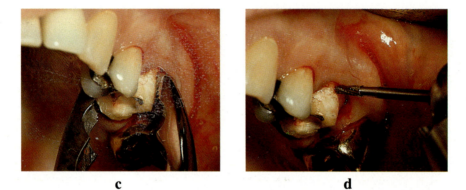

Fig. 10-22, a-f. a, X-ray of a maxillary first molar scheduled for extraction. **b,** Clinical view. **c,** The tooth is first luxated with an elevator, followed by a forcep as shown here. **d,** As the tooth did not respond to luxation attempts, it was decided to remove the crown and work directly with the root complex. **e,** Crown removed. **f,** Root complex sectioned mesiodistally, separating the palatal root from the buccal roots.

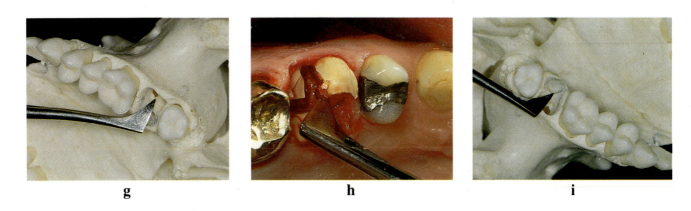

g

h

i

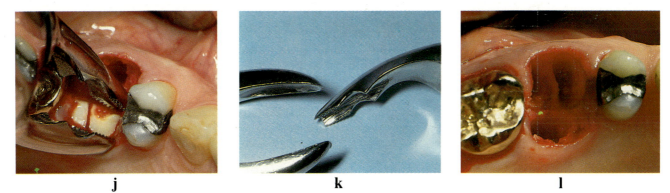

j

k

l

Fig. 10-22, g-m. g, The palatal root will be used as a fulcrum by the large Cryer as this instrument elevates the buccal root(s). **h,** Since the elevator would not disengage buccal roots as one segment, a cut was made between them followed by individual engagement. **i,** Large Cryer applied from the buccal. Heavy forces cannot be used because of the relatively weak support for the instrument. **j,** A forcep using rotational forces is usually more effective than a Cryer elevator in this case. A straight elevator placed into the periodontal ligament in the long axis of the root is also effective. **k,** Serrated beaks of this 150AB forcep on the right provide a solid vise-grip on the root during rotation. **l,** Empty socket. Adjacent teeth were not disturbed during this extraction. **m,** Tooth fragments.

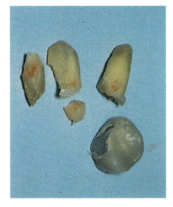

m

Table 10-4. Exodontia Flowchart—Erupted Teeth

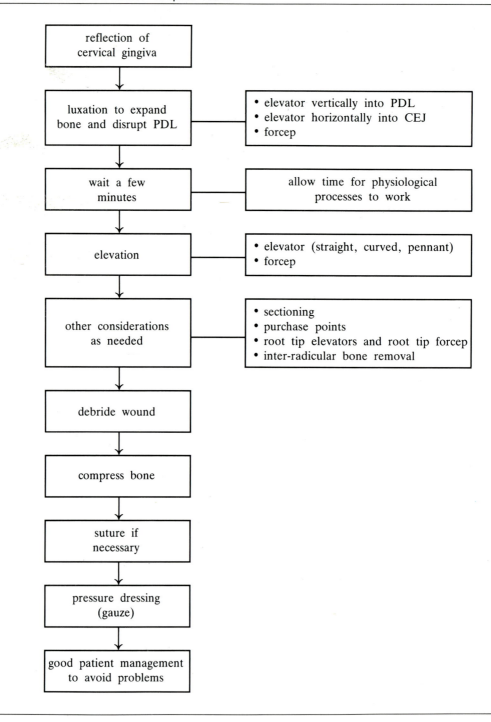

"SURGICAL" EXTRACTION PROCEDURES

When "routine" and "more complicated extractions" cannot be completed with the steps previously described, or when the operator recognizes pre-existing factors that preclude a normal delivery, then flap reflection and bone removal may be indicated to provide adequate visibility and surgical access. This approach is termed "surgical removal."

Table 10-5 includes a list of those anatomic situations that often lead to the necessity of a surgical manipulation to effect removal.

Table 10-5. Conditions that lead to difficulty in exodontia and that may require the "surgical" removal of teeth or roots.

1. Older patient (over 35)
2. Heavy or dense bone, particularly on the buccal
3. Short clinical crowns, especially with evidence of attrition
4. Hypercementosis
5. Divergent roots
6. Sharply curved roots
7. Roots protruding into the sinus
8. Non-restorable teeth with deep caries
9. Teeth with extensive restorations
10. Teeth with large, bulbous roots
11. Roots sharply angulated from the long axis of the crown
12. Non-vital teeth

Flap Design

Mucoperiosteal flaps in these situations are always "full-thickness," but may be envelope, triangular, or trapezoidal. Other characteristics of flaps include:

1. The incision should always be made over bone that will not be removed. This allows bone support for the sutured incision.
2. Flaps should include a full-thickness of mucoperiosteal tissue.
3. The unreflected base of the flap should be wider than the reflected portion of the flap. This insures an adequate blood supply.
4. Flaps should be made large enough to ensure good vision and an adequate area for removal of bone. Releasing incisions are generally made one tooth away from the one involved in the procedure.
5. The operator should be cognizant of all underlying anatomic structures.

In most instances, the operator may feel that sufficient visibility and surgical access is possible with an envelope flap. However, in some instances, a triangular or trapezoidal flap design is utilized for the surgical removal of teeth. Some flap options are shown in accompanying illustrations (Fig. 10-23).

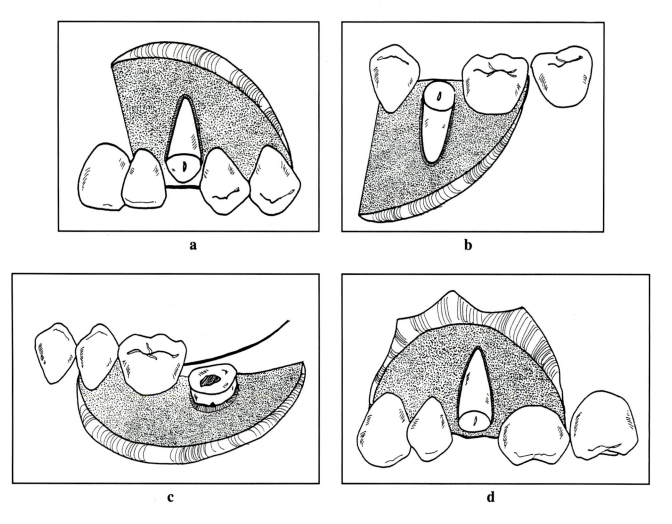

Fig. 10-23, a-d. Flap designs for root access and possible bone removal. Instruments that can be used once this degree of access has been achieved include the straight elevator, forcep (if it can be engaged), and a Crane Pick for insertion into a purchase point on the buccal side next to apical bone.

Bone Removal

The indications and techniques for alveolar bone excision are essential to the dentist performing any exodontia. In certain instances, the capability of some bone removal creates a solution to the tough exodontia problem that would otherwise be impossible. One learns from experience that surgical extraction can often be more conservative than what started as "merely" a forceps extraction. The forceps extraction done with excessive force can cause such morbidity as alveolar bone fracture, exposure of the maxillary sinus wall, and damage to adjacent teeth.

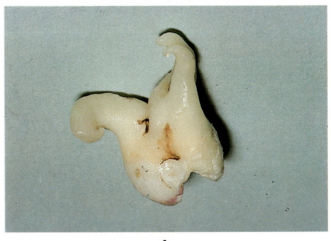

Fig. 10-24, a and b. Examples of teeth that would usually require "surgical" removal (flap reflection and bone removal).

a

b

When excising bone, certain principles in the care and handling of bone must be followed. The reader should refer to these in Chapter 1. The excision of bone for the removal of teeth is usually accomplished from the buccal aspect or inter-radicularly, although it may also be from interproximal areas. Very rarely is lingual bone removed.

Table 10-6 lists root retrieval techniques that the operator should consider after having made the decision to reflect a flap. It is adapted from Peterson, LJ. *Contemporary Oral and Maxillofacial Surgery*, 1988, The CV Mosby Co.

Table 10-6. "Surgical" approach to Retrieving Roots

1. Attempt to reseat the forcep under direct visualization, hoping at this point to increase the mechanical advantage without having to resort to bone removal.

2. Grasp a bit of buccal bone under the buccal beak of the forcep to obtain better control of the tooth.

3. Wedge a straight elevator into the periodontal ligament space to displace the tooth or root coronally.

4. Remove bone on the buccal of the root. The width of buccal bone that is removed is essentially the same width as the root in a mesiodistal direction. In a vertical direction, bone can be removed about one-half to two-thirds the length of the tooth root.[2] In fact, some authors even suggest that bone can be excised to the apex, if necessary, for hypercementosis or severe dilacerations.[3,4,5] This reduces the amount of force necessary (with either an elevator or forcep) to remove the tooth. This approach pertains to all teeth except mandibular third molar impactions. They are handled somewhat differently because of the broad, expansive shelf of bone on their buccal side.

5. If, after this amount of buccal bone removal, the tooth is still difficult to extract, a purchase point can be made in the root with a bur at the most apical portion of exposed root. An elevator such as the Crane pick is used to elevate or lever the tooth from its socket.

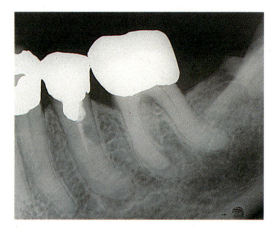

Fig. 10-25, a. The second premolar of this 60-year-old woman exhibits hypercementosis. It is symptomatic and removal is indicated.

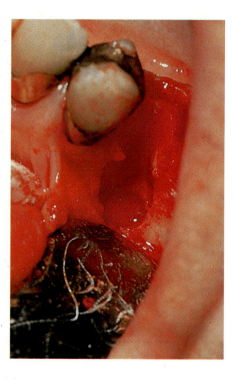

Fig. 10-25, b. As the operator started the procedure, he found that the tooth was extremely brittle. After the crown fracture, small pieces continually gave way in response to elevator application. A releasing incision was made, followed by alternating use of elevator and bur. This degree of bone removal was required to accomplish the extraction.

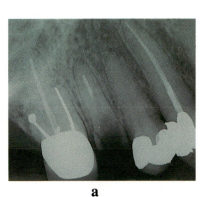

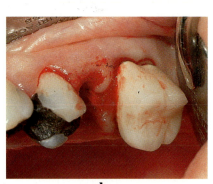

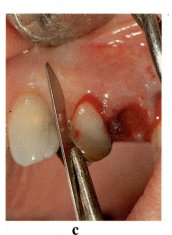

a

b

c

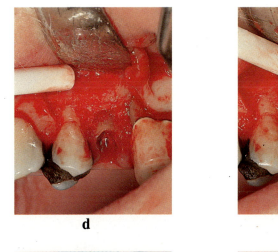

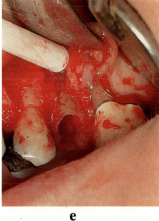

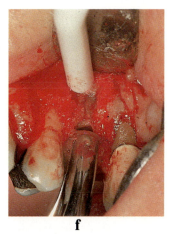

d

e

f

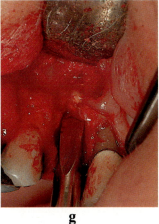

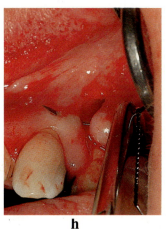

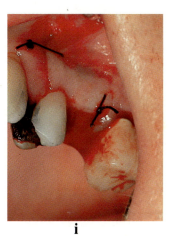

g

h

i

Fig. 10-26. a, X-ray of a second premolar requiring removal. The patient is a 40-year-old woman. **b,** Cervical gingiva has been reflected. Initial application with elevators proved unsuccessful. **c,** A triangular flap was reflected to gain access to the root. **d,** Some buccal bone was excised to provide elevator access. **e,** Since the root still did not budge, more bone was removed. **f,** The forcep was applied but the root fractured at the level of the forcep beak. **g,** Finally, a straight elevator was placed into the lingual periodontal ligament and the operator used reciprocating motion with apical pressure. This had been tried previously without success. This time it worked and the root was removed. **h,** Releasing incision suture being placed. **i,** Sutured case.

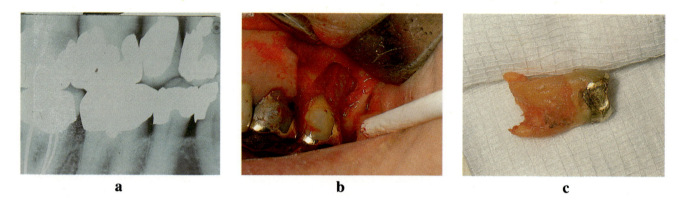

a   b   c

Fig. 10-27. a, Periapical x-ray of a decayed, maxillary second molar indicated for removal. **b**, Since the tooth would not loosen with luxation attempts and because of the weak crown that was predisposed to fracture, the tooth was removed "surgically." **c**, Extracted tooth.

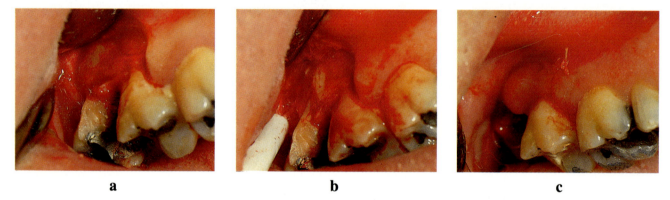

a   b   c

Fig. 10-28. a, Initial extraction attempts resulted in a coronal fracture of this erupted maxillary third molar. **b**, In this "surgical" removal, bone was excised buccal to the roots and the tooth was delivered buccally. **c**, Sutured case.

Fig. 10-29. Some roots do not need to be removed. This asymptomatic root has remained unchanged for nearly 30 years.

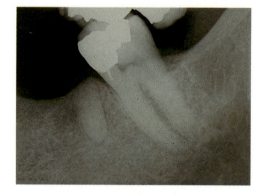

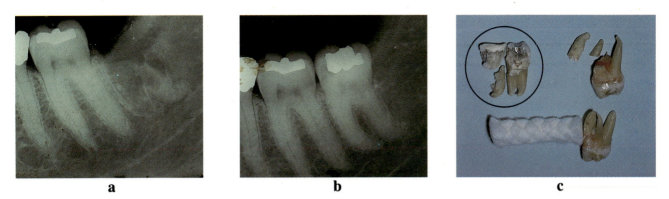

Fig. 10-30. a, This erupted third molar in a 28-year-old man was scheduled for extraction. **b**, During the operation, part of the distal root fractured. Because of the mandibular canal's close proximity, the operator considered leaving the root and informing the patient of this decision, and the reason for it. **c**, With a few more minutes of trying, and some bone removal in the distal elbow area, extrication was finally achieved.

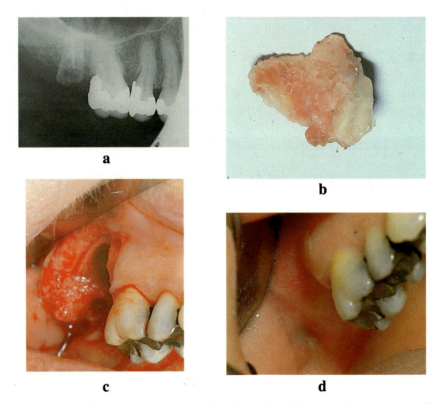

Fig. 10-31. a, This is an x-ray of a fractured second molar of a 55-year-old woman. After unsuccessfully struggling with the extraction through coronal access for several minutes, a triangular flap was reflected. Bone removal and elevator application were alternated until all of the socket wall had been relieved from the buccal and also the distal. **b**, When elevator pressure was increased, the tuberosity fractured. In cases such as this, a careful evaluation must be made prior to removing tooth and bone. Does it involve the hard palate near the greater palatine foramen or will bone lacerate soft tissue as it is removed? Does it involve the distal wall of the sinus or adjacent teeth? If yes, then it may be prudent to suture the flap and consult with a colleague before continuing. Since periosteum lines bone on the lingual aspect, it will most likely remain vital if not removed. A second surgery may be needed for the purpose of removing the tooth by attrition. In this case it was felt that the fracture was small enough to not cause serious problems if removed. **c**, Defect prior to closure. **d**, One month postop.

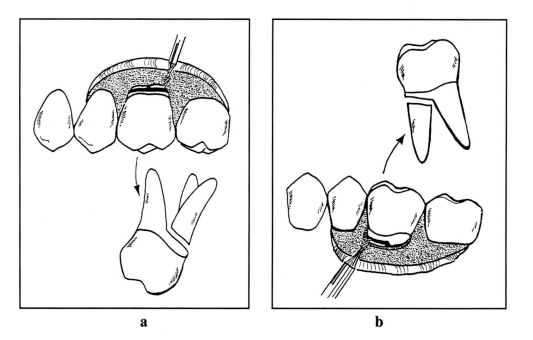

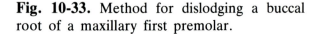

Fig. 10-32, a and b. a, Occasionally with a solid crown on a maxillary molar, the operator will find it useful to section the buccal roots from the remainder of the tooth and remove the palatal root with the crown. This would usually be classified as a "surgical" extraction since a flap would need to be reflected and bone removed at least to the furcation level. Then more bone would most likely need to be removed to expose enough of each buccal root for forcep placement. It is possible that the buccal roots could be removed with elevators only. **b,** The same principle can be put to use on lower molars.

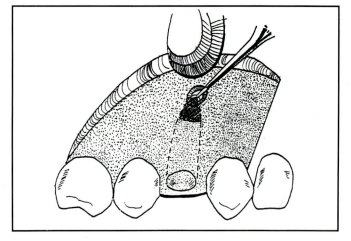

Fig. 10-33. Method for dislodging a buccal root of a maxillary first premolar.

When to Leave a Root

On occasions, it is better to leave a root than to remove it. When would this be the case? Consider the following instances:

1. The root is suspected to be on the verge of entering an anatomic space.
2. It is thought that further instrumentation would cause damage to adjacent anatomic structures.
3. There is uncontrolled bleeding.
4. Removal would require an inordinate amount of bone excision.
5. Patient fatigue that could involve pain, TMJ stress, and emotional distress.
6. Doctor fatigue that could result in inefficiency or impaired judgment.
7. An extended period of time for the surgery – even without obvious fatigue.
8. The root is minimal in size (less than 4-5 mm), vital, undislodged, and without pathology.

In the event a dentist chooses to leave a root behind, the patient must be informed of the occurrence and the reasons for the decision. Documentation of the situation should be recorded in the patient's chart. Fractured roots of healthy teeth over which a clot forms and subsequent healing takes place usually maintain vital pulp tissue and remain asymptomatic. Root tips or other tooth fragments that violate anatomic spaces may or may not precipitate pathology and annoying symptoms but they are definitely more of a risk and a concern. They may or may not need to be removed. Generally a consultation with another dentist or with an otolaryngologist is recommended.

Total Attrition

As a last resort, the operator may choose to "dust away" certain roots rather than leaving them or continuing to attempt their removal. This is especially true if it is suspected that future problems might occur if the roots are left.

Table 10-7. Exodontia Flowchart—"Surgical" Removal

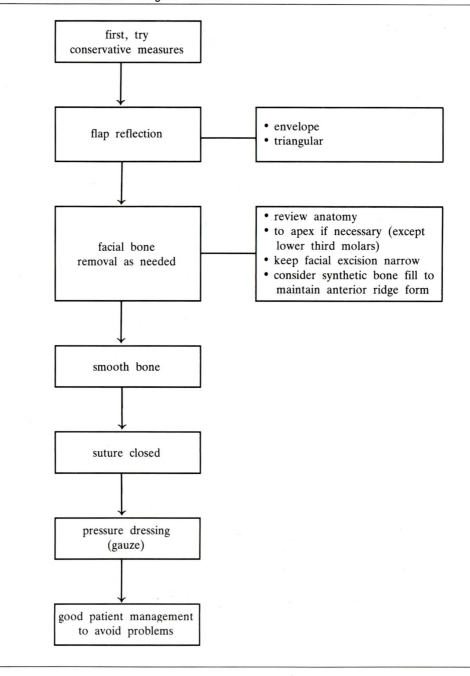

CLINICAL CASES
Case 1
Removal of Crowded Mandibular Bicuspids

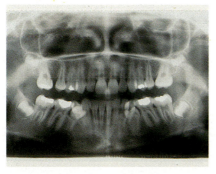

a

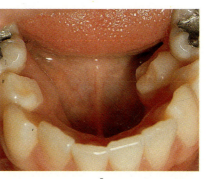

b

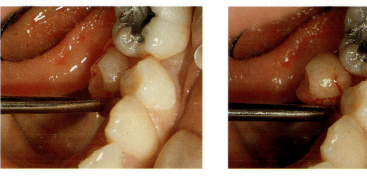

c

d

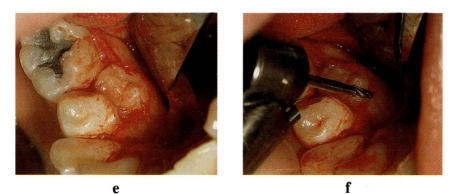

e

f

Fig. 10-34, a-f. a, Panoramic x-ray. **b**, Preoperative clinical appearance. **c**, After cervical gingival reflection, the left tooth is carefully luxated. **d**, Removal. **e**, Reflection of a triangular flap (releasing incision mesially) for access to the tooth on the right. An envelope flap may have been sufficient. **f**, Since attempts at luxation and elevation were unsuccessful, some bone is about to be removed with a bur. This surgical highspeed handpiece is designed not to force air into the surgical field.

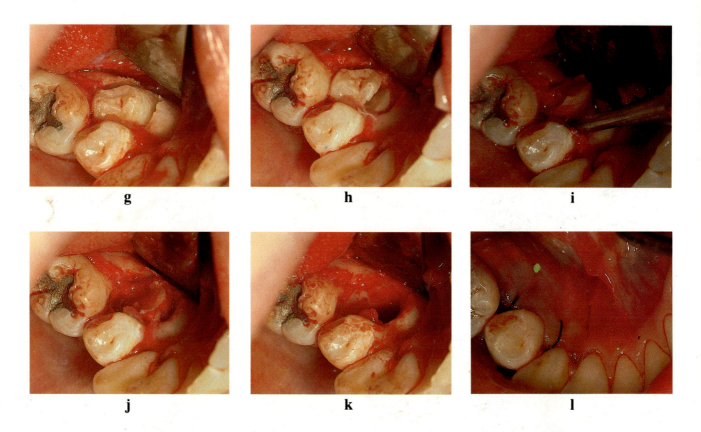

g

h

i

j

k

l

Fig. 10-34, g-m. g, Bone removal. **h**, Sectioning was necessary. **i**, A 301 elevator was used to fracture the tooth in two parts. **j**, Root segment ready to be elevated from the socket. **k**, Empty socket. **l**, Sutured case. **m**, Extracted tooth and tooth fragments.

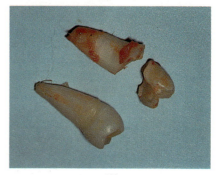

m

Case 2
Supernumerary Removal from Palate

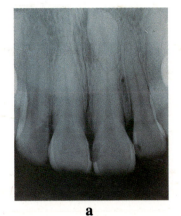

a

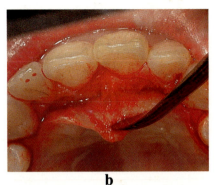

b

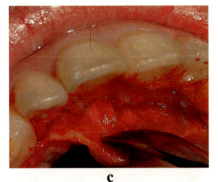

c

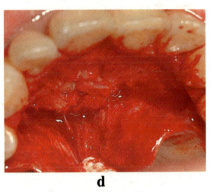

d

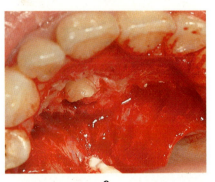

e

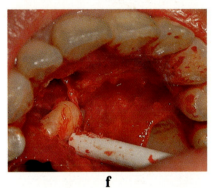

f

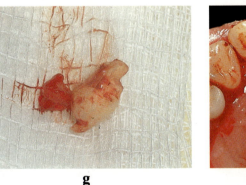

g

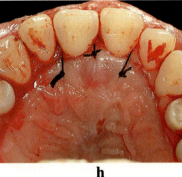

h

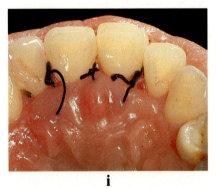

i

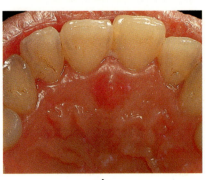

j

Fig. 10-35, a-f. a, Periapical x-ray showing presence of a supernumerary tooth. The actual location of the tooth can be determined by palpation, occlusal x-ray, and a comparison of periapical x-rays taken at different angles. **b,** Beginning of palatal flap reflection. **c,** Continued reflection showing connection of incisive canal structures with underside of flap. **d,** Broadened reflection after incision of incisive nerve and vasculature. These are terminal nerves and vessels that do not usually cause problematic dysesthesia or bleeding. **e,** After some bone removal, enamel of the supernumerary crown is exposed. **f,** Additional bone removal and sectioning (if needed) helps facilitate removal. **g,** Excised tooth. **h,** Palatal soft tissue is readapted, sutured, and pressed into place for a few minutes to initiate adhesion. **i,** Five day postop. **j,** Seven day postop.

Case 3
Multiple Extractions for Immediate Overdenture

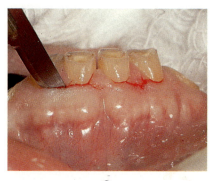

a

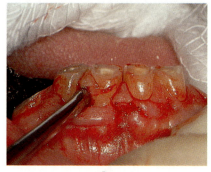

b

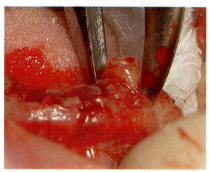

c

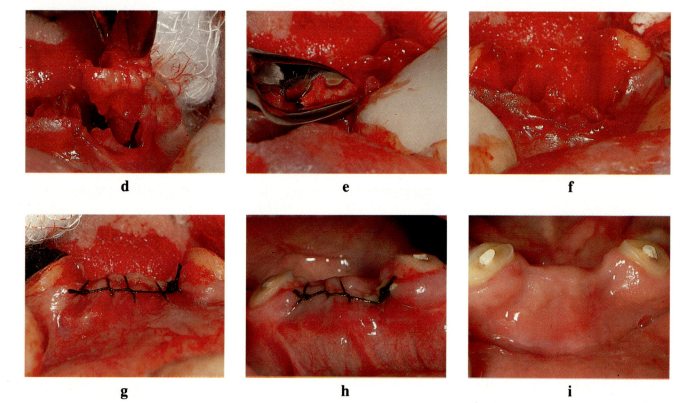

d

e

f

g

h

i

Fig. 10-36. a, Diseased papillae are being excised with a linear incision that touches the facial surfaces of the teeth to be removed. The same type of incision is made on the lingual. **b,** Teeth to be removed are luxated. Luxating adjacent teeth and compressing soft tissue are not contraindicated in this instance since both will be removed anyway. **c,** Teeth are luxated, elevated, and removed with a forcep. **d,** Even with good technique, bone still may fracture and be dislodged with the teeth. **e,** Bone is selectively removed and smoothed with rongeurs, burs, and bone files. When the operator feels the bone through soft tissue with a gloved finger and it is not sharp, then closure may take place, regardless of whether or not sockets are open. **f,** Visual inspection of bone. **g,** Closure with continuous lock sutures. **h,** Five day postop. **i,** Two week postop.

References

1. Phillip G. *Ogram System of Exodontia*. Dallas, Tx; 1991.

2. Peterson LJ. *Contemporary Oral and Maxillofacial Surgery*. St. Louis, Mo: CV Mosby Co; 1988.

3. Costich ER, and White RP. *Fundamentals of Oral Surgery*. Philadelphia, Pa: WB Saunders Co; 1971.

4. Hooley JR, and Whitacre RJ. *A Self-Instructional Guide to Oral Surgery in General Dentistry*. 2nd ed. Seattle, Wa: Stoma Press Inc; 1980.

5. Cogswell WW. *Surgery of the Oral Cavity and the Technique of Controlled Tooth Division*. Portland, Or: Sawyers Inc; 1959.

Suggested Reading

Howe GL. *Minor Oral Surgery*. 3rd ed. Bristol, England: John Wright and Sons Ltd; 1985.

Chapter 11

Simplifying the Removal of Impacted Third Molars

INTRODUCTION

Third molar surgery can be easy or difficult, depending on several factors: patient age, temperament, and health; depth and angulation of the tooth; and knowledge and experience of the operator. Actually, the first and foremost concern is whether or not the tooth is indicated for removal. If it is, then the primary care dentist should plan to perform the operation or refer it to someone else.

The purpose of this chapter is to clarify the indications for removal and then to review factors that help to insure a successful operation. We will reduce third molar surgery to its basic components, thus allowing the dental surgeon to more accurately predict the intrasurgical and postsurgical outcome. It will broaden the operator's comfort zone, increase the range of treatment available to patients in a given practice, and decrease the incidence of negative sequelae sometimes associated with this procedure.

In order for third molar surgery to proceed smoothly, the dentist must be proficient in three areas. These are **case selection, patient management, and operative technique.** This chapter then, is divided into three sections, each addressing one of these topics.

DIAGNOSTIC CRITERIA
Case Selection

Third molars should be evaluated regularly, starting in the mid-teen years. There are several reasons why third molars need to be removed, but there are also reasons why they should *not be* removed (Table 11-1). Some of the most important considerations, however, go beyond a list of indications and contraindications. These points are covered throughout this chapter.

Table 11-1. Third-Molar Removal

Indications for Removal

1. Insufficient space
2. Malposition
3. Pathologic resorption (2nd or 3rd molar)
4. Orthodontic considerations
5. Pericoronitis
6. Need for the tooth in another area (transplantation)
7. Periodontitis
8. Carious involvement
9. Idiopathic symptoms
10. Preceding restorative or prosthetic appliances
11. Presence of a cyst or neoplasm
12. Traumatic injury (fracture through the socket)

Contraindications for Removal

1. Sufficient space for normal eruption
2. Compromised health status
3. Third molars needed as abutments
4. Asymptomatic impactions without pathology in patients over 30-35 years of age—where potential surgical trauma outweighs benefits from removal
5. Patient declines surgery

From Koerner KR. *Clinical Procedures for Third Molar Surgery*. PennWell Books, 1986.

Age and Morbidity

The factor that relates most significantly to surgical difficulty and complications is age. The time in a patient's life at which third molar surgery is least difficult to perform and which results in the least morbidity is when the roots are approximately two-thirds formed. This opinion has been substantiated by an NIH Health Consensus Development Conference, and is now recognized throughout the dental community. At that point in a patient's anatomical development, there is the least likelihood of surgery-related problems. Roots are straight and short, bone is relatively soft, the inferior alveolar nerve is generally not in close proximity to root apices (almost eliminating alveolar nerve paresthesia as a complication), healing is rapid, and downtime from the procedure is not usually a serious matter. In addition, root development has forced the tooth occlusally to the degree that bone removal is minimized, precluding the need for extensive hard tissue excision. The existence of a partial root also prevents revolving of the crown during removal.

Still, the operation should not be recommended indiscriminately. One diagnostic approach for lower third molars has been suggested by Ricketts that helps eliminate surgery for those patients in whom the teeth may indeed have room for eruption.[1] He reasons that since jaw formation and third molar crown calcification are both complete by about age 16, an undistorted radiograph can be used to predict future relationships. A line is drawn along the occlusal plane and another along the ascending ramus: the distance between the point where these two lines intersect and the distal surface of the second molar represents the space available for the third molar (Figure 11-1).

Fig. 11-1. A tracing of the lateral headplate of a 19-year-old male shows Ricketts' method of evaluating the space available for the third molar. The point at the intersection of the external oblique ridge with the molar occlusal plane serves as a reference. The portion of the third molar ahead of that point suggests the space that is available. When 50% of the tooth is ahead, the chances for eruption are considered to be 50%. Here the chances are about 30%, and the molar is caught slightly behind and below the second molar. (From Ricketts RM. Studies leading to the abortion of lower third molars. *Dent Clin North Am.* 23:393, 1979.)

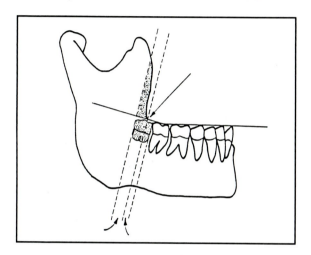

If the alveolar bone in this area is flat far enough distally to accommodate a tooth, then surgery may not be necessary. One should realize that there must not only be sufficient space for the occlusal aspect of the tooth, but for axial surfaces as well. Third molars that have soft tissue over their distal height of contour, which may even include an operculum over the distal marginal ridge, are not good candidates for a lifetime of service in the mouth. They are difficult to keep clean and are predisposed to decay, pericoronitis, and periodontitis. Unless there is going to be firm gingiva at a fairly normal cervical level, the teeth should be removed at an early age to avoid inevitable problems. An exception might include patients who want to see how long they can maintain these partially erupted teeth, especially if there is good home care.

Generally, this surgery is much easier in younger people. By examining radiographs from persons in their late teens (when root development is not yet complete), we find a two millimeter follicle around unerupted teeth, a periodontal ligament that is about .25 mm wide, roots that are not yet formed, and well trabeculated, elastic bone. If the tooth is unerupted, it can be removed by merely creating a "pathway" for delivery.

Fig. 11-2, a. There is sufficient space for this mandibular third molar to have erupted normally, contraindicating removal. Attached gingiva surrounds the tooth.

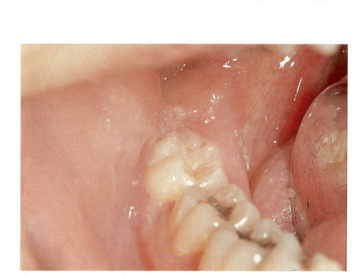

Fig. 11-2, b. This third molar could be classified as a soft tissue impaction, as gingiva is well over the height of contour distally to include an operculum over the distal marginal ridge. Although an operculectomy may preclude future periodontal problems, the tooth is still at high risk for eventual decay and periodontitis. It lacks attached gingiva on the distal—one of the most difficult areas in the mouth to keep clean. The tooth should be considered for removal.

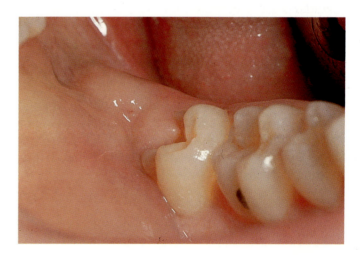

Fig. 11-2, c. A more obvious indication for extraction, this third molar in a 23-year-old obviously does not have room for normal eruption. Decay and infection are inevitable. It is intermittently symptomatic.

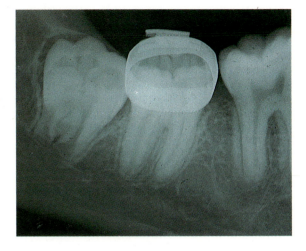

Fig. 11-3, a. This radiograph shows that there is insufficient space for this tooth to ever be functional in the arch. When is the best time for removal? Now—as prospects are lowest for surgical morbidity. The roots are approximately two-thirds formed.

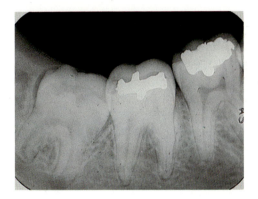

Fig. 11-3, b. Same as above, only the roots are about three-fourths formed.

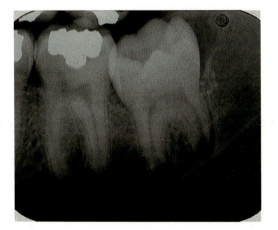

Fig. 11-3, c. Even though the possibility of inferior alveolar nerve paresthesia should be presented to the patient, its likelihood is negligible. Superior and inferior lamina dura of the mandibular canal can be seen as they cross the tooth, there is no distinct radiolucency of tooth structure where the canal traverses past the root, and there is no constriction or flaring of the canal. The operator can be reasonably certain that the canal lies in buccal cancellous bone. It is merely superimposed radiographically on the tooth. (See Fig. 11-4.)

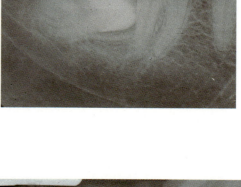

Fig. 11-3, d. This tooth is past its "prime" for removal, yet because the patient is still under 25 years of age, complications will be minimal. The risk of paresthesia should be explained to the patient although it would not be expected (See Table 11-2).

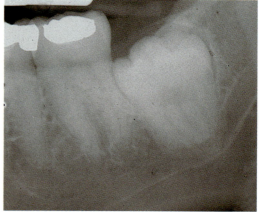

Fig. 11-3, e. Canal deflection increases the risk of what would most probably be a temporary sensory alteration of the nerve.

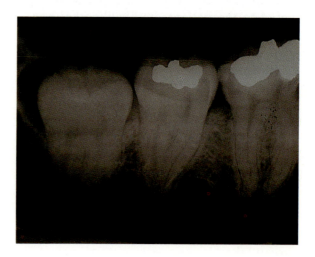

Fig. 11-3, f. A widened follicle space (over 2 mm on a periapical film or 3 mm on a panoramic) suggests that this developmental tissue be submitted for histological examination.

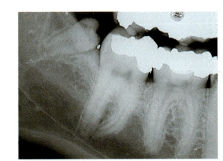

Fig. 11-4, a. Supernumerary that was noticed two years following the removal of four third molars.

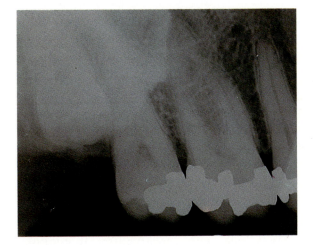

Fig. 11-4, b. Same as **a.** above, only in a different patient.

Later in life, the anatomic situation changes dramatically. Bone gradually fills in around the crowns of unerupted teeth, completely encasing them in bone; the periodontal ligament closes in tightly around the root; roots can develop dilacerations and hypercementosis; and bone becomes more dense and in some cases, even sclerotic. When these teeth are removed at more advanced ages, sectioning forces can be transmitted directly to investing bone with the potential of serious trauma instead of having these forces dissipate into elastic tissues as with younger individuals (see Figure 11-5). Table 11-2 compares intraoperative and postoperative complications with third molar surgery as they relate to age.

Fig. 11-5, a. Maxillary complete bony impaction in a 46-year-old man. The tooth has long been arrested in its eruption. The two millimeter developmental sac found in younger people has disappeared and been replaced with bone. The quarter of a millimeter periodontal ligament space has atrophied. Bone is generally more dense and less trabeculated than it was 25-30 years ago.

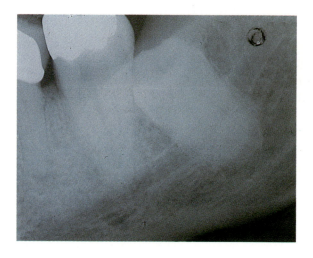

Fig. 11-5, b. Mandibular third molar in a 60-year-old woman.

Table 11-2.

Surgical problems increase linearly with age. In comparing patients under 25 with those over 35, we find:

During surgery	under 25	over 35
excessive bleeding	1.5%	9.7%
traumatic case	1.2%	9.7%
nerve encountered	0.6%	7.3%
lingual plate fracture	0.6%	3.9%
fractured root	3.6%	7.3%
average operating time	8 minutes	18 minutes
After surgery	**under 25**	**over 35**
excessive pain	4.8%	20.3%
excessive swelling	2.4%	17%
excessive trismus	0.9%	10.6%
excessive ecchymosis	0.9%	7%
hematoma	0.3%	4.2%
dry socket	7.6%	17%
lingual nerve paresthesia	0.6%	1.8%
inferior alveolar n. paresthesia	1.2%	9.7%
prolonged healing	1.8%	10.6%
postop visits	1.5	3.5
days before asymptomatic	10.6	34.1

Adapted from Bruce RA, Frederickson GC, and Small GS. Age of patients and morbidity associated with mandibular third molar surgery. *JADA.* 101:240, 1980.

Occasionally, we see patients in their 30s and beyond who have unerupted third molars. If these teeth are asymptomatic, without evidence of pathology, and with no discernable communication with oral fluids, then they should not necessarily be removed. Instead, the general consensus is that they should be periodically reevaluated. Radiographs should be taken to reexamine their status every 3-5 years. If they are problematic, only then should removal be considered. Certainly there is a diagnostic "grey area" in dealing with third molar removal that will continue to be subjective and dependent on clinical and radiographic findings, as well as the operator's experience level and judgement.

All in all, this seems to be a reasonable and pragmatic approach to third molar removal that combines logic with conservatism. It minimizes complications, particularly one that is the dentist's nemesis, inferior alveolar nerve paresthesia. In view of the concern over this nerve and also the lingual nerve, a brief discussion of these anatomic entities follows.

Lingual Nerve

Lingual nerve paresthesia with third molar surgery is not common. According to a study by Bruce,[3] occurrence is 0.6% with patients under 25 years of age, rising to 1.8% in those over 35. Anatomically, the nerve is usually lingual to the third molar—about two millimeters down from the alveolar crest and 0.5 millimeters from the lingual plate (see Fig. 11-6a). Kiesselbach's research[4] revealed, however, that 17% of the time, this nerve is at or above the crest of the ridge (see Fig. 11-6b).

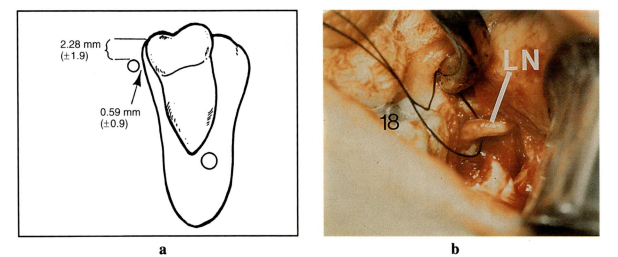

a   b

Fig. 11-6, a and b. a, Frontal view of the left third molar region showing the mean horizontal and vertical distances of the lingual nerve from the lingual plate and alveolar crest. **b,** The lingual nerve has been identified, blunt dissected from adjacent soft tissues, and surrounded by a silk suture during a mandibular third molar surgery procedure. (From Kiesselback JE, and Chamberlain JG. Clinical and anatomic observations on the relationship of the lingual nerve to the mandibular third molar region. *J Oral Maxillofac Surg.* 41:565, 1984.)

Considering both of these possible locations of the nerve, we can then list ways that the nerve can be injured during or after the surgery. Whether it is located high or low, it can be injured by:

1. Making the distal incision too far lingually (nerve high)
2. Perforating lingual tissue with a periosteal or apical elevator (nerve high)
3. Lacerating with the bur when removing occlusal bone (nerve high) or distal bone (nerve high or low)
4. Lacerating when making a section cut through the tooth (nerve high or low)
5. Pinching with forcep beaks if lingual tissue inadvertently included (nerve high or low)
6. Fracturing the lingual plate and tearing or stretching lingual tissue (nerve high or low)
7. Pinching or stretching tissue when removing the follicle (nerve high)
8. Perforation with a suture needle (nerve high)
9. Tearing when incorrectly treating a dry socket (nerve high)

The incidence of lingual nerve trauma from needle injury (during the injection) is low. In these cases, the nerve usually heals in several weeks, although the damage can be permanent. The nerve is 10-15 times larger than the diameter of the needle, making it unlikely that the needle will sever the nerve. Damage is more likely from penetration of the central arteriole or the epineural blood vessels, causing hemorrhage, hematoma, and then metabolic and functional disturbances from associated compression. Prolonged compression or infection can lead to scarring, fibrosis and permanent damage.[2]

Inferior Alveolar Nerve

Inferior alveolar nerve paresthesia is more common with third-molar surgery than lingual nerve paresthesia. The rate is 1.2% with patients under age 25, 2.4% in the 25-35 age group, and 9.7% in those over 35.[3] When the surgery is performed in patients with roots two-thirds formed (the ideal time), paresthesia incidence is negligible.

As demonstrated by cadaver studies in which wires were drawn through the mandible, the canal usually traverses buccally in cancellous bone. Occasionally it can be found on the lingual or even between the roots of third molars. Radiographically it can be found apical to third molar roots or superimposed across the roots.

Paresthesia is more common when the canal containing the nerve is found in a notch or groove on the buccal, lingual, or at the apex of a third molar. In rare cases, third molar roots will actually encircle the canal. When this occurs, the nerve can be stretched and/or torn as the tooth is removed unless great care is taken. These anatomic anomalies are often discernable radiographically.

Sometimes the tooth will rest passively against the nerve and vasculature of the canal with no bony interface. When this happens, almost any degree of luxation can bruise the nerve as the tooth is removed. Disruption of the inferior alveolar artery can also cause paresthesia from ischemic effects on the nerve.

The vast majority of inferior alveolar nerve paresthesias are temporary, but the time span is unpredictable. Even the most gentle encounter can sometimes result in unexpectedly long-lasting consequences. That is why informed consent is so important.

Figure 11-7 illustrates several signs of intimate proximity between the canal and a third molar. Table 11-3 lists factors that predispose inferior alveolar nerve paresthesia.

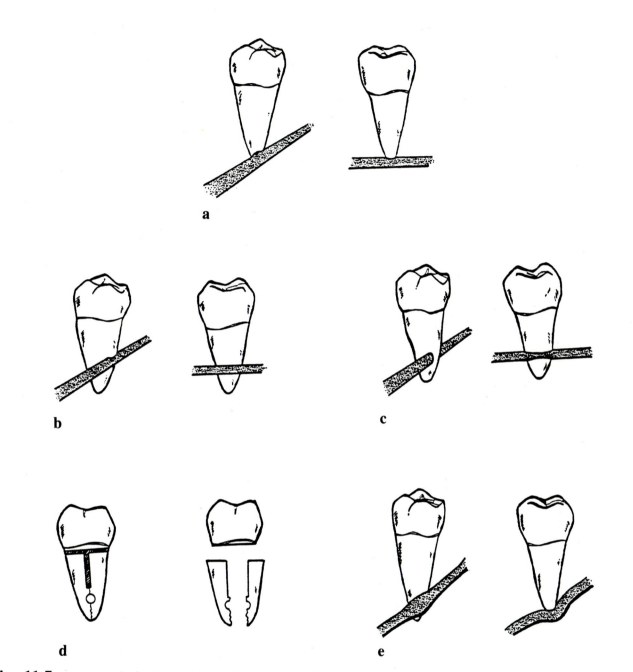

Fig. 11-7, a-e. a, Apical notching. The root is limited in its apical development by cortical bone surrounding the mandibular canal. **b,** Grooving. Similarly, a groove is notched into the root as it forms around the canal during development. In both apical notching and grooving the x-ray reveals a radiolucency along the tooth because of a decreased density of tooth structure in the area occupied by the canal. **c,** Perforation. In this instance the canal is totally enveloped by tooth structure. The canal appears constricted in the middle of the tooth. In a, b, and c the white lamina dura of the canal (upper and lower borders) are lost when it enters tooth structure. **d,** Surgical technique. If perforation is suspected and the tooth must be extracted, the crown should be removed followed by root sectioning from anterior to posterior. **e,** Flattening (left) and deflection (right). These both indicate intimate proximity to the root that may result in bruising and subsequent dysesthesia as the root is luxated and removed.

Table 11-3. Factors that relate to inferior alveolar nerve paresthesia. (From Koerner KR. *Clinical Procedures for Third Molar Surgery.* PennWell Books, 1986.)

The following factors increase the average incidence of paresthesia (from 4-5% on up).

Preoperatively:

1. Loss of the canal's lamina dura*

2. Radiolucent band across the tooth (grooving)*

3. Radiolucency at the root apex (apical notching)*

4. Narrowing or constriction of the canal across the tooth*

5. Deflection of the canal*

6. Flattening of the canal*

7. Deep impactions, especially horizontal

During surgery:

1. Visualization of the canal

2. Excessive bleeding

3. Bone removal near the apex

The following factors decrease the average incidence of paresthesia (from 4-5% down to 0-2%).

1. Roots not completely formed

2. Canal traversing at a level beneath the apex

3. Patients under 25

*More discernable with periapicals than panoramic radiographs

---

If, despite the operator's best surgical effort, paresthesia occurs, it should be monitored with periodic scheduled visits (such as once a month) until the final disposition is clear. At each appointment, the location of sensory deficit should be described as to how the size of the involved area changes and how the surface sensations change (no feeling, prickly, etc.). Generally, patients gradually regain normal feeling within a few weeks to a few months.

Permanent numbness generally occurs from stretching, tearing, or cutting the nerve, although even a severed nerve has the potential to regenerate under certain circumstances. If normal nerve function has not returned within two years, it is unlikely that it will return at all—even though there are rare exceptions.

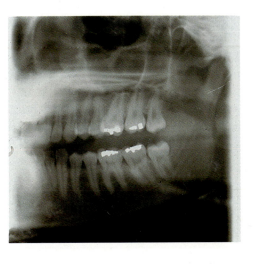

Fig. 11-8, a. Partial panoramic film of a 25-year-old woman. Note the mandibular third molar. Four third molars were scheduled for removal.

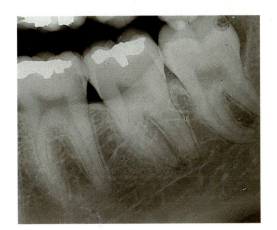

Fig. 11-8, b. Radiograph of tooth #32.

Fig. 11-8, c. Extracted teeth—#17 and #32. When the root tip of #32 fractured, the operator made an attempt with a root tip pick to remove it. After a few minutes and without success, the distal part of the socket suddenly filled with blood. The decision was made to leave the root tip and inform the patient.

When the woman returned five days later, the right side of the lower lip was profoundly numb. Arrangements were made to follow the case by examining her once a month until the situation was resolved. One month later, numbness had changed to a prickly feeling that was aggravated by touch. She was assured that this was a normal part of the healing process. At two months, she returned to say that the lip was back to normal except for a small spot near the midline—about one centimeter in diameter. By three months, feeling in the lip was totally back to normal.

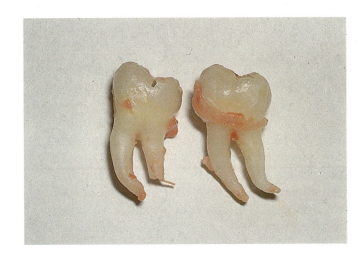

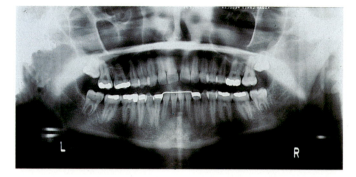

Fig. 11-9, a. Radiograph of a 28-year-old woman. All four third molars were removed. The lower ones exhibited pericoronitis and the upper right third molar was erupting buccally into the cheek.

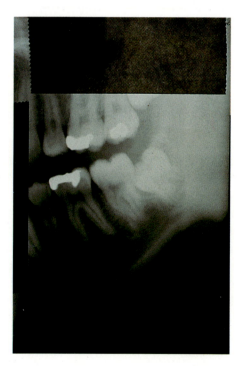

Fig. 11-9, b. Some minor complications included visualization of the inferior alveolar nerve on both sides and fat from the facial space entering the surgical site on one of the maxillary procedures. This picture shows the operator's attempt to photograph the neurovascular bundle. (Also see Fig. 11-60e.)

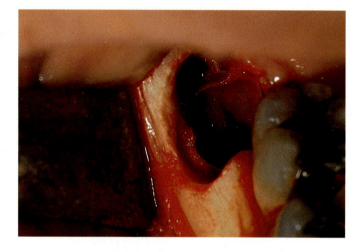

Fig. 11-10, a. This inferior quality panoramic film was borrowed from another dentist to save the patient (an 18-year-old man) expense and radiation exposure prior to the removal of four third molars. The operator should have taken another film.

Fig. 11-10, b. During the surgery, the crown was removed and the root complex was sectioned through the bifurcation. The distal half was removed followed by elevation of the mesial half. After the mesial portion was elevated, it snapped back down into the socket when the elevator was removed. It turned out that the canal passed directly between the distal and mesial roots with the mesial root hooking inferiorly around the canal. The elasticity of the canal explained why the tooth was pulled apically. No paresthesia resulted.

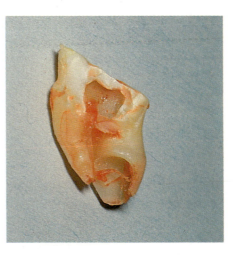

Fig. 11-11. This woman had four impacted third molars removed. After the anesthesia wore off, normal feeling returned to the lip and chin. Three days later she returned, complaining of bilateral paresthesia. She is pointing to the part of her face that feels numb. Normal feeling returned after another 3-4 days. The author's explanation is that of rebound edema affecting an anatomically vulnerable nerve. Oral steroids had been administered for three days, beginning preoperatively. Without the anti-inflammatory medication, paresthesia probably would have started sooner and lasted longer.

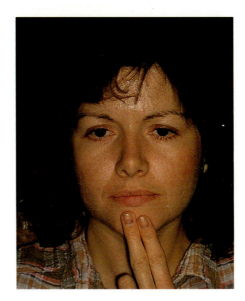

PATIENT MANAGEMENT

The topic of patient management covers all those influences aside from case selection and technique that make the surgery go smoothly; influences that insure that the patient will be satisfied during and after the procedure. Good patient management enhances the doctor-patient relationship, thus providing protection from patient dissatisfaction and potential liability. It includes the following:

1. A good chairside manner that instills patient confidence

2. Informed consent

3. Accepting only those cases that are within the doctor's ability and "comfort zone"

4. A fairly accurate prediction of how long the procedure will last

5. Having a staff that is knowledgeable regarding the procedure

6. Preventing or mitigating anxiety, pain, swelling, trismus, dry sockets, and infection with the proper use of medications

7. A knowledge of how to deal with postoperative healing and potential complications that may occur

A doctor who is knowledgeable and prepared for a procedure will transfer that impression to the patient. That is not to say that every problem can be anticipated. It does mean, however, that the surgery is within the operator's skill level and that the tooth will be removed in a reasonable length of time. If complications occur, they will be dealt with carefully and professionally.

Informed Consent

Informed consent, usually to include the signing of a form for that purpose, is mandatory. Patients have the right to know why the tooth should be removed and what inherent risks are associated with the procedure. If, after being informed, the patient refuses surgery, that right should be respected and duly noted in the record. A sample consent form is shown in Table 11-4.

Table 11-4.

Consent Form for Third Molar Surgery

The surgical procedure that is to be performed has been explained to me and I understand the nature of my condition and of the proposed treatment. I also understand what health risks exist if the procedure is not done, such as pain, infection, decay, damage to other teeth, and a more difficult surgery as I get older.

I agree to the administration of local anesthesia and other therapeutic measures as discussed that may be necessary for my comfort, safety, and well-being.

I realize that occasionally there are complications with this surgery and the medications. The more common complications include pain; swelling; bleeding; dry sockets; limited mouth opening; infection; bruising and discoloration of the skin; and temporary numbness and/or tingling of the lip, chin, gums, cheek, teeth, or tongue.

In some cases, even with the utmost care there can be referred pain to the ear or neck; stiffness of the neck and facial muscles; changes in the bite and temporomandibular joint (TMJ); nausea; allergic reactions; bone fractures; injury to adjacent teeth; delayed healing; and permanent numbness of nerves in the facial area. Sinus complications which may occur from the removal of upper teeth include a root tip or tooth in the sinus, or development of a lingering opening into the sinus from the mouth which could require sinus treatments following this surgery.

Medications given during or after surgery may cause drowsiness and a lack of awareness and coordination which could be increased by the use of alcohol or other drugs. I am aware that I should not operate any vehicle or hazardous devices while taking such medications and at least 24 hours after taking them or until recovered from their effects.

I know that some of the above-mentioned complications can be avoided or reduced by carefully following the doctor's instructions. I have had an opportunity to ask questions about the procedure and aspects related to it and have had them answered to my satisfaction. This is my consent to surgery.

_____   _____
Signature   Date

_____
Guardian (if a minor)

Medications

Table 11-5 reviews medications that contribute to an uneventful procedure.

Table 11-5. Suggestions for Medications that Can Be Used with Third Molar Surgery.*

1. **Anti-inflammatory medication:**
   - First choice—oral non-steroidal anti-inflammatory agents
   - Second choice—oral steroids (more effective but slightly greater risk of complications)

2. **Oral sedation:** usually a benzodiazepine-based regimen.

3. **Nitrous oxide:** optional.

4. **Topical anesthetic:** this is especially advantageous for palatal injections. Use a cotton swab applied with pressure.

5. **Long-acting local anesthetic:** pain from bone removal is strongest 3-5 hours after surgery. Long-acting anesthetic helps patients through this period of most intense pain.

6. **Systemic antibiotics as indicated:** *Primary indications:* pre-existing infection, compromised health conditions, anatomic space contamination. *Other considerations:* difficult or traumatic case, steroids, local standard of care.

7. **Meds to prevent dry socket:** most commonly Gelfoam™ with a tetracycline-containing solution.

8. **Sterile saline irrigation:** It enhances healing and lessens the incidence of dry sockets.

9. **Pain meds as needed:** generally moderate analgesics.

*Review the health history and contraindications.

Communication with the Patient

Table 11-6 outlines possible contacts with the patient before, during, and after third molar removal, especially as these pertain to the dentist's assistant and receptionist.

Table 11-6.

There are several "patient-office contacts" that need to be addressed in planning for third molar surgery. They are:

1. Several days or weeks before the procedure
2. The day before surgery
3. The day of surgery
   - immediately prior to surgery
   - during the operation
   - immediately following surgery
   - the evening of that same day
4. Five-to-seven days postoperatively

At any one of these times, interaction with the patient or guardian can be through the doctor, the receptionist, or the dental assistant.

1st Contact: Several days or weeks before the procedure

Persons involved: doctor, receptionist and dental assistant
- Review the health history
- Take x-rays
- Discuss possible sedation options
- Inform the patient about possible complications
- Have patient read and sign the consent form
- Clarify the fee and payment method
- Schedule the procedure
- Arrange for a prophylaxis, if indicated
- Review diet restrictions

2nd Contact (telephone): The day before surgery

Person involved: doctor, receptionist
- Confirm the appointment
- Review necessary medications
- Call prescriptions to pharmacy
- Review diet restrictions

3rd Contact: Immediately prior to surgery

Persons involved: receptionist, dental assistant
- Help the patient feel calm
- Review food intake that day
- Check all paperwork
  - informed consent signed
  - insurance information received
- Prepare instruments and supplies for surgery
- Monitor office asepsis

During the operation

Persons involved: doctor, dental assistant, optional 2nd assistant

- Surgical procedure

Immediately following surgery

Persons involved: doctor, receptionist, dental assistant

- Review medications - give prescriptions if not already done
- Give written postoperative instructions and supply of gauze
- Make an appointment for postop check/suture removal
- Give doctor the patient's telephone number

The evening of that same day (telephone)

Person involved: doctor

- Doctor calls the patient

4th Contact: Five to seven days postoperatively

Persons involved: doctor, dental assistant

- Evaluation of healing
- Suture removal (if nonresorbable sutures were placed)
- Dry socket treatment if needed
    - pack placement may necessitate another visit for removal
    - patient may need an irrigation syringe

This kind of involvement and support in the office will help make third molar surgery an uneventful and problem-free part of a practice.

Postoperative Instructions

Proper care of the mouth by the patient following surgery can reduce the incidence of complications and speed the healing process.

Before leaving the office, the patient (or one responsible for helping the patient to return home safely) should be given the following:

- Written postoperative instructions including an appointment for suture removal and information on how to receive after-hours emergency care
- Any necessary prescriptions for postoperative medication
- A supply of gauze pads to last for a few hours (with instructions to get more if needed)

Table 11-7 gives an example of postoperative instructions that can be given to the patient.

Table 11-7.

Care Following Dental Surgery

To insure rapid healing and to avoid complications that could be both harmful and painful to you, please follow these instructions carefully.

1. **Bleeding.** To prevent unnecessary bleeding, maintain gentle pressure over the surgery site(s) by biting on gauze. You have been given a supply of gauze pads. If more are required, they can be purchased at a drug store or supermarket. A tea bag which has been moistened and wrapped in a piece of gauze is also effective. Pressure should be continued for 1-2 hours or until most of the bleeding has stopped. Change the packs every 15-20 minutes or when saturated. It is not unusual to have some slight oozing for up to 24 hours.

   Rest today and keep your head slightly elevated. Do not engage in physical activity since this stimulates bleeding.

2. **Medications.** Unless you already have your medications, pick them up very soon and take as directed. Frequently with oral surgery a long-acting local anesthetic is used—especially if bone was removed. This prevents pain, but may also prolong numbness for up to 24 hours. Take a pain pill when you first feel discomfort. If you took sedative medications (such as Valium), do not drive for at least 24 hours after surgery.

3. **Eating.** It is important to get adequate nutrition after surgery to help the healing process. Just drink liquid food supplements or juices and eat soft foods today. Progress to more solid foods as healing progresses.

   If wisdom teeth were removed, your jaw is temporarily weaker than before surgery. For that reason, you should not chew forcefully or engage in contact sports for 5-6 weeks. To do otherwise could cause a bone fracture.

4. **Rinsing and Brushing.** Do not rinse for the first day after surgery since this could dislodge the blood clot. This could lead to a dry socket. After 24 hours, rinse with warm salt water (1/2 teaspoon of table salt in 8 oz. water) 3-4 times a day for 4-5 days.

   Besides rinsing too soon, other actions that can contribute to dry sockets are smoking and using a straw.

5. **Ice Packs.** To help prevent swelling, ice packs should be applied to the face adjacent to the surgery sites. This is especially important if bone was removed. To the extent possible, apply for periods of 20 minutes on and 5 minutes off until bedtime on the day of surgery. Ice is not particularly useful after the first day.

   With most oral surgery, swelling peaks at about 48 hours and then goes down. Significant swelling beyond this time period could indicate infection. If this occurs, call the dentist.

6. **Postoperative Check-up.** The surgery site needs to be examined to make certain that healing is progressing normally. In addition, sutures may need to be removed. The date and time for your follow-up visit is:_____ .

7. **Unforeseen Complications.** If you suspect any problems with healing, do not hesitate to call the office or the doctor at home. These telephone numbers are:

Office: _____   Home: _____

Sometimes patients develop allergies to medication, infection (foul taste, unusual or prolonged swelling), and dry sockets (throbbing pain 3-5 days after the procedure). These and other potential problems are treatable if brought to the doctor's attention.

In our office, we are doing everything we can to make your surgery as painless and uneventful as possible. However, what you do following your surgery is important too.

SURGICAL TREATMENT
Last Minute Review

The actual removal of impacted third molars is a straightforward process. However, there are a few things that must be considered prior to beginning any procedure. Among these are:

- **Is the tooth indicated for removal?** (Refer to the first section of this chapter.)

- **Is the patient manageable and willing to have it done the way you want to do it?** (Refer to the second section of this chapter.)

- **How old is the patient?** If too young (roots not formed), perhaps you should wait until the roots are closer to 2/3 formed. If over 25 years old, it may be a reason for the generalist to refer to a specialist—particularly if it is quite deep.

- **How deep is the tooth?**

  Lower: If the occlusal surface is below the cementoenamel junction of the second molar and/or if it is mostly in the ramus and not in the body of the mandible, then it will probably be quite difficult, especially in an older person.

  Upper: If it is higher than the cementoenamel junction of the second molar and/or if there is more than one millimeter of bone over the occlusal surface, it will probably be a hard one. High distoangulars with fully formed roots usually present more problems than verticals.

- **What is the patient's facial form?** Is it tapering or compact in shape? If tapering, the procedure will be much easier than if compact. A face that tends towards being more compact will have shallow mucobuccal folds, a high floor of the mouth, shallow palatal vault, and low zygomatic arch— all contributing to difficult access and a higher incidence of complications.

- **From radiographic and clinical inspection, is it within your comfort zone?**

Mandibular Third Molar Impactions

Now that you have decided to perform the extraction, we will discuss the six steps necessary to complete the procedure. They are:

1. Reflect a flap that gives good access and visibility.
2. Selectively excise bone around the crown as needed.
3. Luxate at appropriate intervals.
4. Section tooth structure when appropriate.
5. Elevate and remove the tooth or portions of it until the socket is empty.
6. Debride and close the wound.

Step 1—Reflect a flap that gives good access and visibility.

There are many flap variations for third molar impaction surgery, and all are described in dental literature. Only three will be shown here. Two are envelope designs and one includes a releasing incision.

Fig. 11-12. This picture depicts a very conservative envelope flap extending to the mesiobuccal line angle. Normal cervical reflection is used for an erupted tooth. It gives good access for a shallow impaction. The most critical part of it is the distal incision. It must be angulated from the middle of the second molar's distal surface laterally toward the external oblique ridge. Its length depends on clinical circumstances and need. The lateral angulation fulfills three requirements: It avoids the lingual nerve; it keeps the incision on bone rather than dropping off into an anatomic space to the lingual; and it helps the operator stay clear of the retromolar artery.

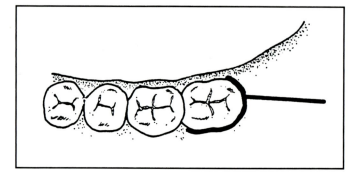

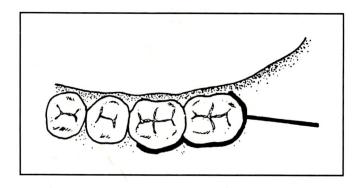

Fig. 11-13. The flap shown here differs only in that the anterior component is extended to the mesial line angle of the first molar (instead of just the second molar) for increased access in deeper cases. At times it may be necessary to excise a wedge of tissue from the distal of the second molar instead of simply making the linear incision, such as when there is redundant tissue that the operator feels has the potential of causing a pseudo pocket following the procedure. This wedge must be conservative in order to avoid lingual nerve proximity.

Fig. 11-14. This triangular flap design has a releasing incision, thus providing access for even the deepest bony impaction. The releasing component begins near the second molar's mesiobuccal line angle about one-third of the way into the papilla. It extends downward at a slight oblique angle stopping just short of the mucobuccal fold. This forward angulation helps preserve tissue health and vascularity in the corner where vertical and horizontal cuts meet. Stopping short of the mucobuccal fold eliminates the risk of nicking the facial artery or anterior facial vein that traverse across the inferior border of the mandible. Starting the vertical component on the distal side of the papilla where there is usually a broader band of attached gingiva helps avoid possible periodontal defects such as a dehiscence over the second molar root at the incision line. At the end of the procedure, this flap will be repositioned from where it was lifted up, thus preserving tissue health around the second molar.

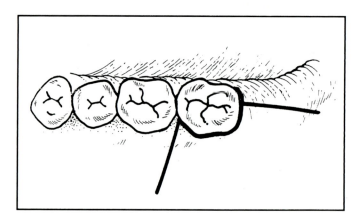

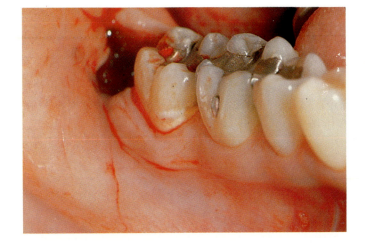

Fig. 11-15, a. A simple, conservative envelope flap. Mesially, it extends to the mesiobuccal line angle of the second molar.

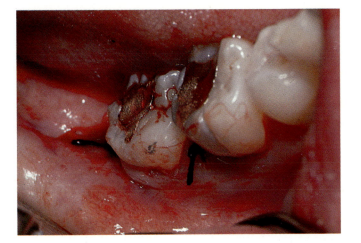

Fig. 11-15, b. An extended envelope flap. Mesially, it includes the papilla and extends to the mesiobuccal line angle of the first molar.

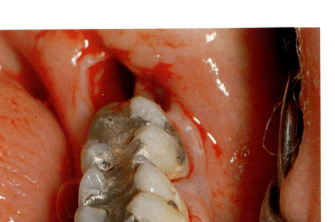

Fig. 11-15, c. Another extended envelope flap—with a tear on its mesial aspect—buccal to the first molar. When this occurs it means that either the operator was not careful enough with the flap or that a triangular flap design should have been used.

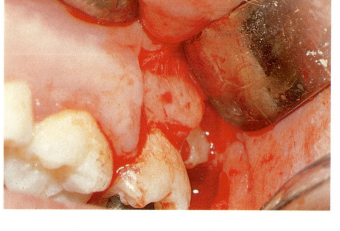

Fig. 11-15, d. A triangular flap showing the releasing incision.

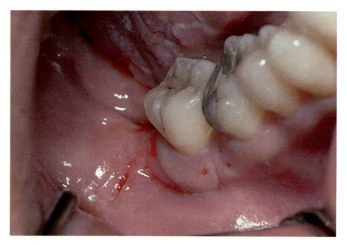

Fig. 11-15, e. Five-day postoperative look at a healing triangular flap.

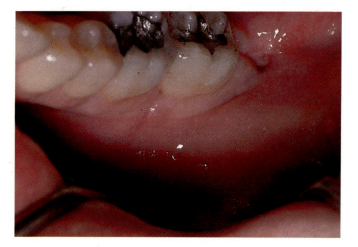

Fig. 11-15, f. Another five-day postoperative view.

Step 2—Selectively excise bone around the crown as needed.

Enough bone should be excised to give the operator sufficient surgical access for sectioning and elevator placement. Bone removal is done in two ways:

- shelf removal to get a "straight on" view of the tooth, and

- troughing with a fissure bur along the buccal surface of the tooth to cut a narrow trench approximately down to the bifurcation.

Initial bone removal may include excision of bone from the **superior, buccal, distal, and at times even the mesial surface,** depending on the depth and angulation. It eliminates the "higher" bone, mainly around the crown. For example:

> **mesioangular (most common type):** superior, buccal, distal bone
>
> **horizontal:** superior, buccal bone
>
> **vertical:** superior, buccal, distal bone
>
> **distoangular:** superior, mesial, buccal bone

Very rarely is bone ever removed from the lingual in this conventional American approach. In other parts of the world, dentists often use a lingual split-bone technique but its disadvantages are that it is done with mallet and osteotome, generally requires general anesthesia, and has a higher incidence of lingual paresthesia.

Troughing usually extends down to the bifurcation level, particularly with mesioangular, distoangular, and vertical impactions. By creating this narrow trough, strength of the mandible is maintained, purchase for an elevator is made, and some of the bony encasement around the tooth is lessened. It is largely at the expense of the buccal surface and extends apically to the area of the bifurcation although the bifurcation is never actually visualized.

The distal excision is not usually as deep as the buccal trough and must be carefully executed because of the lingual plate's close proximity. It is made mainly to remove that lip of bone over the tooth's distal height of contour.

Step 3—Luxate at appropriate intervals.

Luxation is accomplished with the appropriate elevator or, if the tooth is superior enough, a forcep. This movement tests for adequate anesthesia, expands bone, and partially disrupts the periodontal ligament. In many cases, it will lead directly to elevation and removal.

Step 4—Section tooth structure when appropriate.

Sectioning eliminates the need for any additional bone removal, thus preserving the strength of the jaw. Section cuts into a tooth are often made with a 702 or 1702 bur followed with fracture by a 301 elevator. A cut does not need to extend all the way through the tooth on the lingual to be effective. In fact, it is recommended that it stop short of the tooth's lingual surface by as much as one millimeter out of deference to the lingual nerve.

A longitudinal cut through the center of a tooth may enter the furcation area with no untoward effects. The elevator used to separate the tooth into segments should be placed as deep into a section cut as possible to maximize contact area and efficiency. Sectioning options for various angulations are presented in Figures 11-16 through 11-20. These illustrations are from Koerner K R. *Clinical Procedures for Third Molar Surgery*, PennWell Books, 1986.

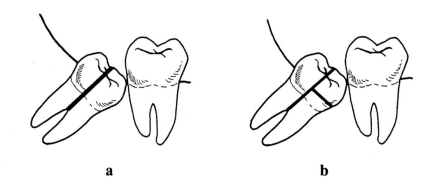

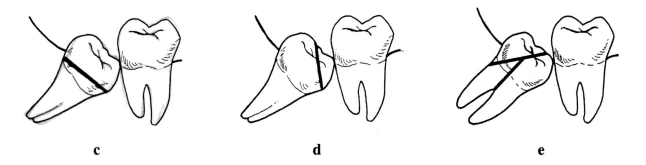

Fig. 11-16. Mesioangular impaction. **a,** Through furcation. **b,** Through furcation, then section mesial root. **c,** Section off crown. **d,** Mesial slice. **e,** Distal slice through furcation, then section mesial root.

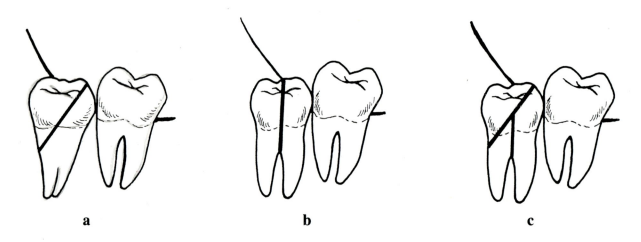

Fig. 11-17. Vertical impaction. **a,** Diagonal section cut. **c,** Through furcation. Remove the least curved root first. **c,** Diagonal section cut, then through furcation.

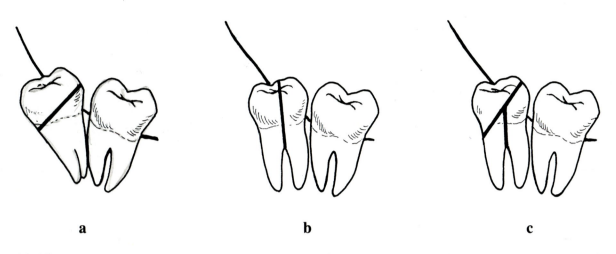

Fig. 11-18. Distoangular impaction. **a,** Diagonal section cut. **b,** Through furcation. **c,** Diagonal cut, then through furcation.

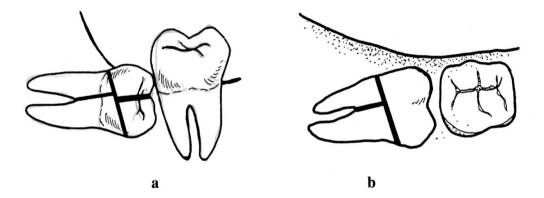

Fig. 11-19. Horizontal impaction. **a,** Conventional crown cut then separate roots. **b,** Rotated 90 degrees.

Fig. 11-20. Transverse impaction. Section crown, then move the root into the crown space.

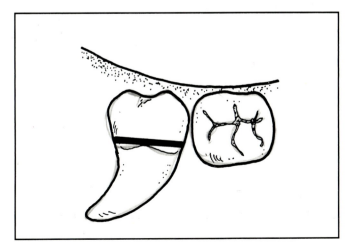

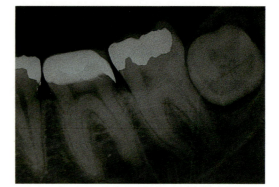

Fig. 11-21, a. Radiograph of a transverse impaction that seemingly could have the crown facing either buccally or lingually.

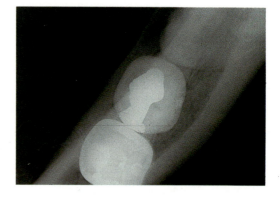

Fig. 11-21, b. Another periapical film oriented in an occlusal manner reveals that the crown is facing the thin lingual plate, as is usually the case.

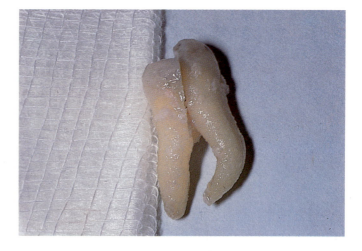

Fig. 11-22, a. Extracted vertical impaction showing how the section cut divided the tooth for removal.

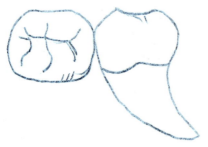

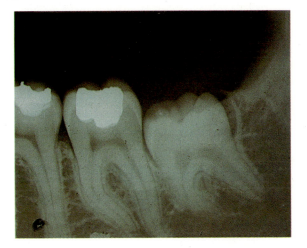

Fig. 11-22, b. Another example of sectioning to facilitate removal of a tooth that would otherwise be very difficult to extract.

Fig. 11-23, a. Impacted third molar that would normally require sectioning as part of the surgical process.

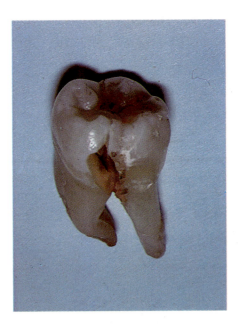

Fig. 11-23, b. Sectioned, extracted tooth with halves placed back in proximity to each other. Because the tooth was sectioned with a straight handpiece (30,000 rpm) the operator found it easier to avoid the dense enamel of the occlusal region.

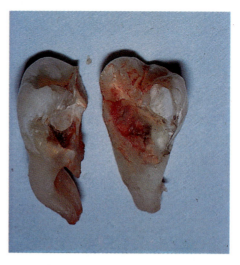

Fig. 11-23, c. Internal view.

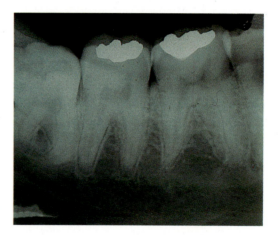

Fig. 11-24, a. Vertical impaction requiring surgical removal.

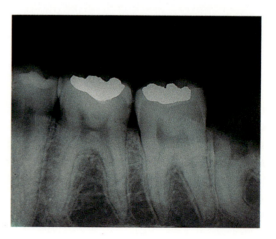

Fig. 11-24, b. The operator removed bone and started sectioning this impaction with a straight handpiece, but the cheek would not stretch enough to allow the bur to divide the tooth through the bifurcation. In a frustrating sequence of events, the crown was lost but the root remained. The distal-most cut on the root shows the best angle the operator could obtain. A surgical high-speed handpiece was then used to make a cut in a more mesial location on the root. After the second cut, the root complex was sectioned and quickly removed.

Fig. 11-25, a. Since this tooth exhibited conical or fused roots radiographically, the operator decided to merely section off the distal portion, thus freeing space into which the remainder of the tooth could be moved.

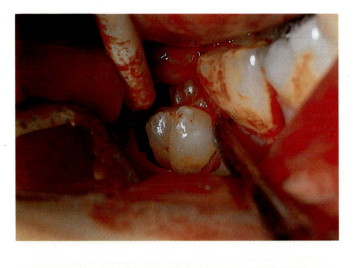

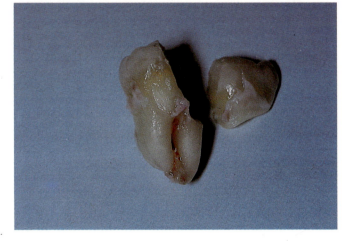

Fig. 11-25, b. Extracted tooth.

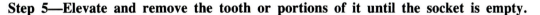

Step 5—Elevate and remove the tooth or portions of it until the socket is empty.

Elevation is usually accomplished with an elevator, although a forcep may be used with shallow impactions. See Chapter 10.

Step 6—Debride and close the wound.

Once a tooth has been removed from the socket, the follicle should also be removed. This applies to impacted teeth only, since partially erupted and erupted teeth will generally not exhibit this developmental tissue. The removal technique usually involves gentle dislodgement with a surgical spoon curette, traction with a surgical suction tip, then grasping and pulling with a hemostat or needle holder. Care should be taken not to traumatize the lingual nerve in the process.

Bone and tooth chips must be cleansed from the surgical site, including along the fold of the flap, to prevent the possibility of inflammatory responses and infection.

The flap is then repositioned, after which mild pressure is applied for a minute or so to eliminate blood and saliva from under the flap and to begin the formation of a fibrin clot. Usually a minimum number of sutures are needed to tack the flap in place. Variations of primary closure (numerous sutures along the distal incision) and secondary closure (0-2 sutures along the distal incision) are used by clinicians. Both are acceptable. The important factors are good tissue adaptation, at least enough sutures to keep the flap in position, and postoperative pressure for clot initiation.

The basic instruments used for removing an impacted third molar are given in Table 11-8.

Table 11-8. Armamentarium

Primary Instruments
1. Surgical handpiece, bur
2. Mouth mirror
3. Surgical suction tip
4. Retractor
5. Periosteal elevator
6. Scalpel and blade
7. Surgical scissors
8. Needle holder
9. Straight elevators, such as 301 and 34S
10. Upper and lower forceps

Back-up Instruments
1. Miller or Potts elevators
2. Cryer elevators
3. Crane Pick or Cogswell B
4. Root tip picks
5. Others according to personal preference

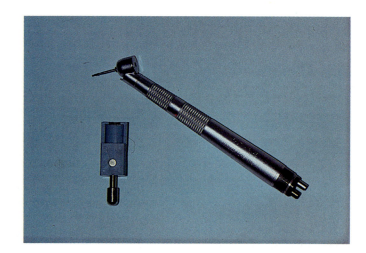

Fig. 11-26, a. Surgical highspeed handpiece. Features include: favorable head angle, fiberoptics, irrigation portal (for water—without air), autoclavability, and head large enough to accommodate surgical-length burs.

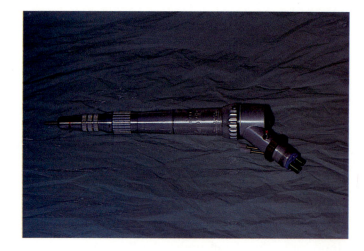

Fig. 11-26, b. Straight handpiece frequently used for impaction surgery. The higher of its two speeds is used (about 30,000 rpm).

Fig. 11-26, c. This handpiece and bur are inappropriate for impactions. The handpiece is a conventional high-speed one that forces an excessive amount of air into the field, predisposing air emphysema. The bur was a 701—too weak for this procedure.

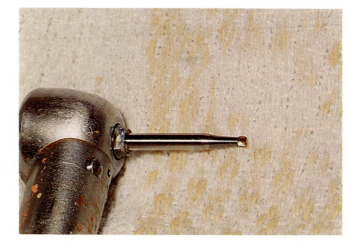

The preceding sequence of steps is illustrated for a mesioangular impaction in Figure 11-27. Figure 11-28 reviews the mandibular horizontal impaction surgery technique.

Fig. 11-27 Surgical technique for a mandibular mesioangular impaction. a, Distal incision from near the external oblique ridge to the middle of the distal surface of the second molar.

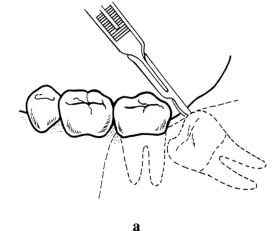

a

Fig. 11-27, b. Overhead view.

b

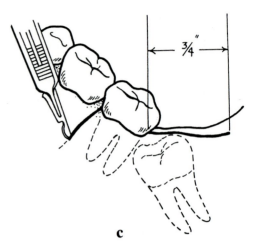

c

Fig. 11-27, c. Harry Archer suggests that the distal part of the incision is generally about three-fourths of one inch long. A releasing incision is being made from the mesiobuccal line angle of the second molar downward, not to extend past the mucobuccal fold.

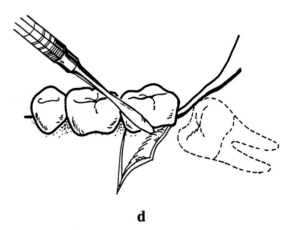

d

Fig. 11-27, d. In this case, the pointed end of a Molt #9 periosteal elevator is being used to lift up the anterior portion of the full-thickness mucoperiosteal flap. Once started, the other end may be used to continue its development. Sometimes a scalpel or scissor may be necessary to dissect fibrous attachments connecting the follicle to the underside of the occlusal aspect of the flap.

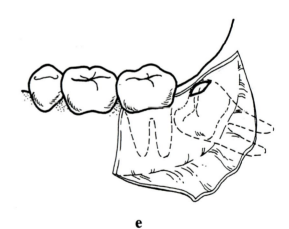

e

Fig. 11-27, e. Full reflection. Note the degree of access.

Fig. 11-27, f. Bone is now being removed from the first of three sides of the third molar—the occlusal.

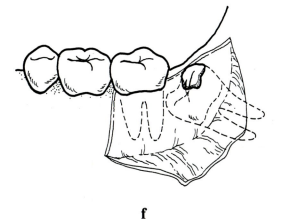

f

Fig. 11-27, g. Next, bone is removed from the buccal surface of the tooth. The buccal shelf is removed down to somewhere between the height of contour and cementoenamel junction to expose the tooth to direct vision.

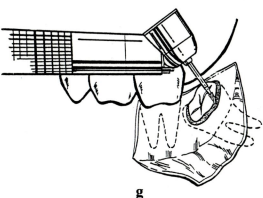

g

Fig. 11-27, h. Distal bone is also removed to remove the lip of hard tissue over the height of contour.

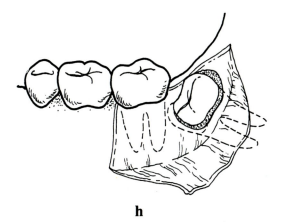

h

Fig. 11-27, i. In this picture, the bur is being used to create a trough along the buccal surface tooth to the depth of the bifurcation. It does not need to extend to that depth on the distal. The width of the trough should not be much wider than the bur itself.

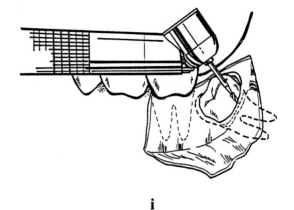

i

Fig. 11-27, j. A section cut has been made in the long axis of the tooth. It may extend to the bifurcation, but generally stops short of the lingual surface in deference to the normal position of the lingual nerve (see section 1 of this chapter). Since a straight elevator will probably be used next to fracture the tooth, this cut should be angled slightly across the tooth, starting somewhat mesial to the buccal groove on the buccal and projecting to a point on the lingual of the tooth that is distal to the lingual groove. The width of the section cut should not be much wider than the bur.

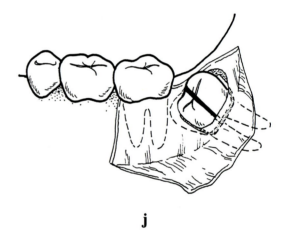

j

Fig. 11-27, k. A straight elevator is inserted deep into the body of the tooth and turned sideways, causing the tooth to break in half. Ideally, the break will split the tooth through the middle.

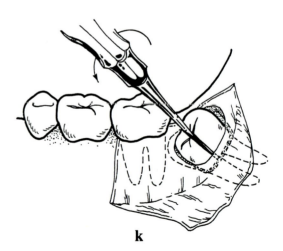

k

Fig. 11-27, l. A wider straight elevator is placed in the buccal trough, and the distal half of the tooth is elevated upward.

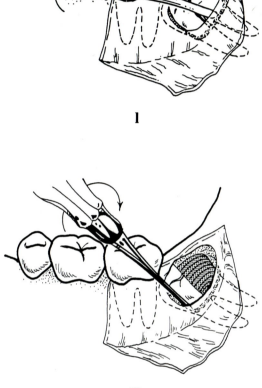

l

Fig. 11-27, m. With the distal half removed, the mesial half can now be rolled upward and even distally (if it is curved).

m

Fig. 11-27, n. The tooth is binding against the second molar.

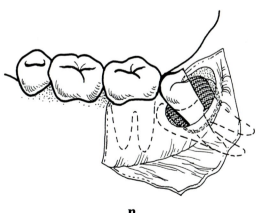

n

Fig. 11-27, o. A "B" cut is made, dividing the mesial half in two, after which the elevator is used to complete severance.

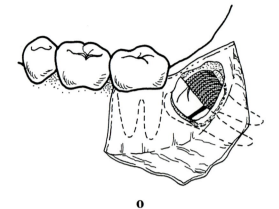

o

Fig. 11-27, p. With the coronal part removed, the elevator is now used to tease out the root.

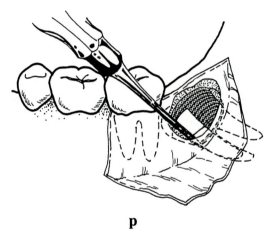

p

Fig. 11-27, q. The follicle was loosened with a surgical spoon excavator, then the suction tip was used to stretch out the loose tissue. It was then peeled away with a hemostat or needle holder.

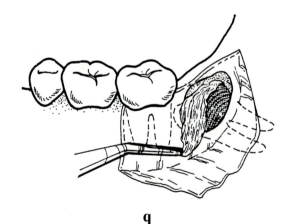

q

Fig. 11-27, r. Two sutures were placed. The first one on the buccal and the second just distal to the second molar, tucking the soft tissue low against the tooth. From Koerner KR. *Clinical Procedures for Third Molar Surgery*, PennWell Books, 1986.

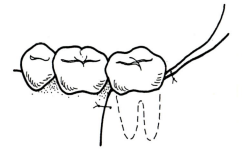

r

Fig. 11-28 Surgical technique for a mandibular horizontal impaction. a, Triangular flap reflection.

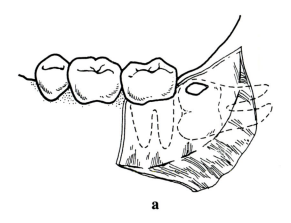

a

Fig. 11-28, b. Bone is removed from the superior and buccal aspects of the crown. The apical extent of bone removal will depend on the depth of the tooth. It will vary from excision down to the buccal groove (deeper teeth) to excision down to the inferior aspect of the crown (more shallow teeth). In this illustration, it is depicted midway between those two levels. Note that no bone is removed from between the second and third molars, nor from the lingual.

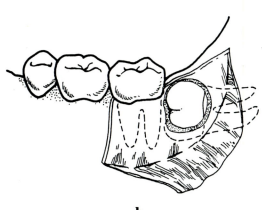

b

Fig. 11-28, c. Bone removal on the superior surface of the third molar is extended posteriorly to expose 4-5 mm of root surface.

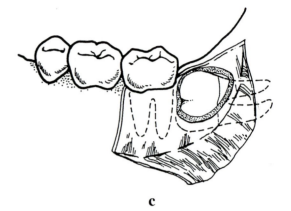

c

Fig. 11-28, d. An "A" cut is made from the superior cementoenamel junction diagonally downward to "just under" the tooth's height of contour. This creates a wedge-shaped segment of tooth that is designed for ease of removal. Once this cut is fractured completely through with an elevator, the operator should attempt to elevate the crown. If it offers too much resistance, a "B" cut can be made as shown. The crown can then be removed in two halves.

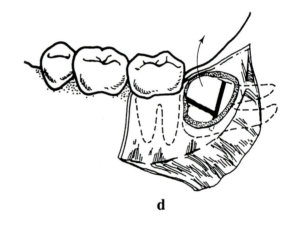

d

Fig. 11-28, e. With the crown out, a purchase point about two millimeters deep is placed in the superior root surface—at least two millimeters from the "A" cut.

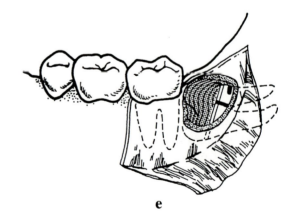

e

Fig. 11-28, f. With distal bone as a fulcrum, the operator can attempt elevation of the root complex with a Crane Pick or Cogswell B. If it does not loosen quickly, the section cut can be made between the roots followed by their removal one at a time.

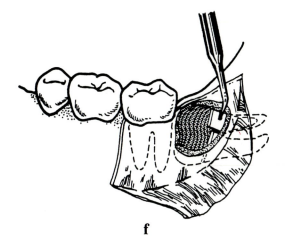

f

Fig. 11-28, g. The inferior root being elevated from its socket.

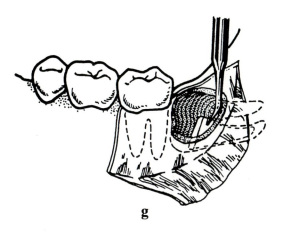

g

Fig. 11-28, h. The empty socket. From Koerner KR. *Clinical Procedures for Third Molar Surgery*, PennWell Books, 1986.

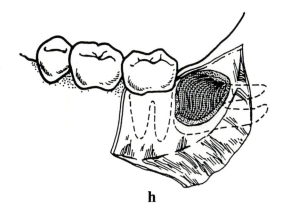

h

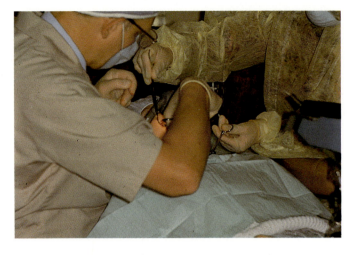

Fig. 11-29. Example of sit-down, four-handed dentistry for impaction surgery.

Fig. 11-30, a. Third-molar removal is much easier in patients with this type of facial anatomy. This man has what might be termed a "tapering" facial form, in contrast to the more "compact" form shown later. With this type, there is excellent access. Roots can be palpated or flaps reflected to teeth apices without encountering the mucobuccal fold. The floor of the mouth is low, putting the tongue and other soft tissues out of the immediate surgical area. The palatal vault, zygomatic arch, and maxillary sinus are high. The mandible's coronoid process does not obstruct visibility of the maxillary tuberosity and third molar with a buccal approach.

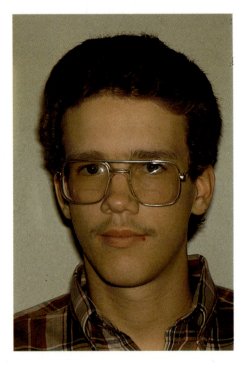

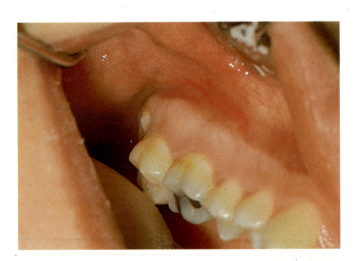

Fig. 11-30, b. Maxillary third molar area on a patient with tapering facial form.

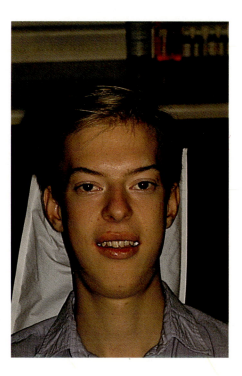

Fig. 11-30, c. Another patient with this type of anatomy.

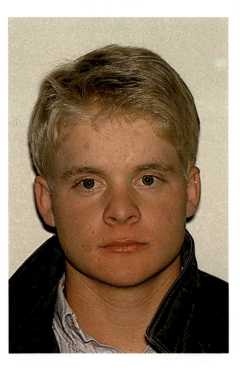

Fig. 11-30, d. Patient exemplifying compact facial form. Pictures are very difficult to obtain on a patient with this anatomy. In the maxillary second molar area, the mucobuccal fold is very close to the free gingival margin.

Fig. 11-30, e. Panoramic film of the patient pictured above. Even though the occlusal surface of the maxillary third molars was near the cementoenamel junction of the second molars (which usually indicates that the surgery will be easy), this case was very difficult.

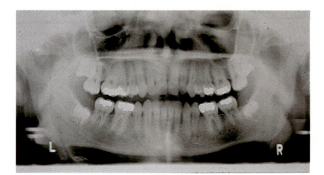

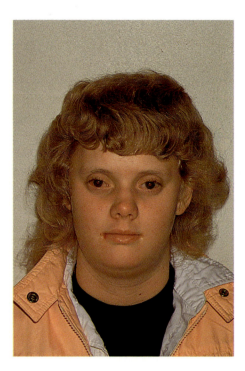

Fig. 11-30, f. Another patient with compact facial form.

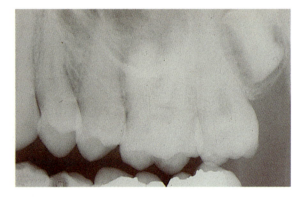

Fig. 11-30, g. Periapical x-ray from the patient shown above. In the process of removal, there was a communication with the maxillary sinus.

Fig. 11-31, a. Periapical x-ray of a surgery to be shown step by step. The patient is 17 years of age.

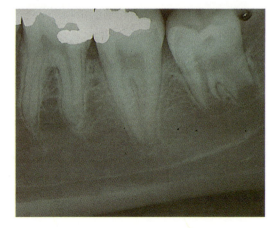

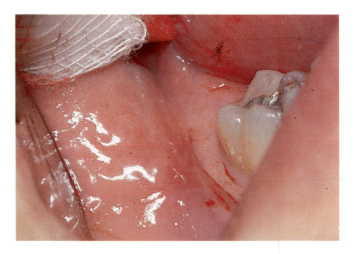

Fig. 11-31, b. Preoperative clinical view.

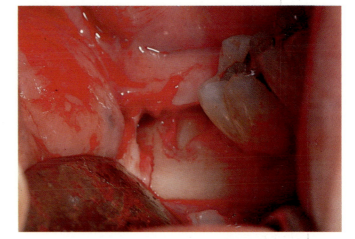

Fig. 11-31, c. Flap reflection showing the degree of tooth impaction in bone.

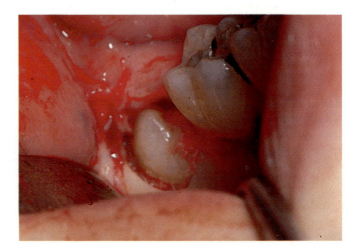

Fig. 11-31, d. Bone removal, including troughing (see text).

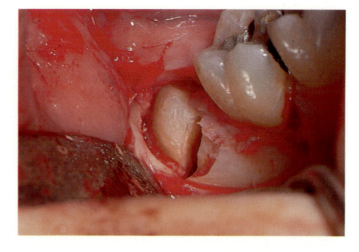

Fig. 11-31, e. Section cut.

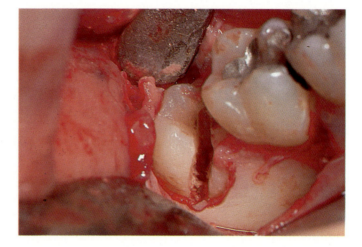

Fig. 11-31, f. Soft tissue retraction to provide a pathway for removal.

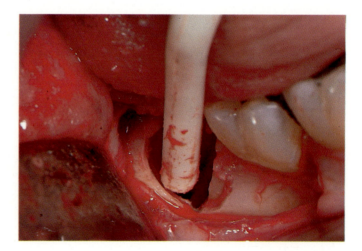

Fig. 11-31, g. Distal half removed. Even though not much of the mesial half is showing, it is easily elevated occlusally and distally.

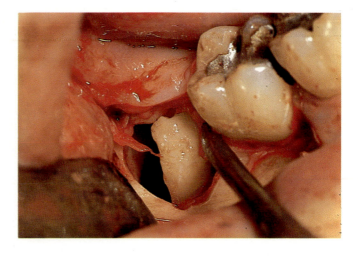

Fig. 11-31, h. Mesial half being elevated. If the second molar is touched at all, it should only be with gentle pressure.

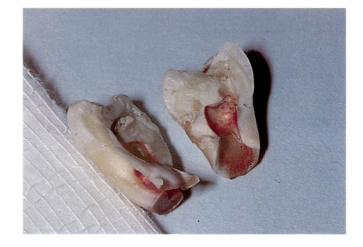

Fig. 11-31, i. Extracted tooth.

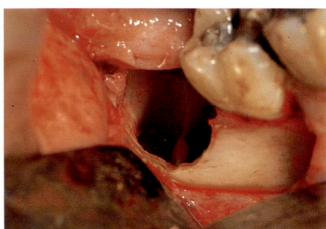

Fig. 11-31, j. Empty socket ready for follicle removal and general debridement.

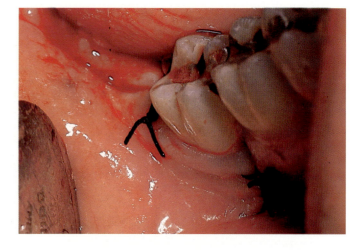

Fig. 11-31, k. Sutured case.

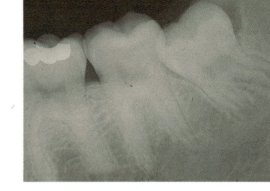

Fig. 11-32, a. Mesioangular impaction to be removed from a 21-year-old woman.

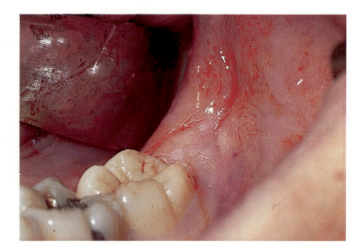

Fig. 11-32, b. Preoperative view.

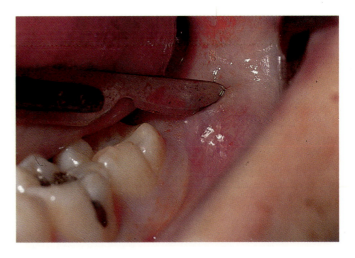

Fig. 11-32, c. Distal incision being made.

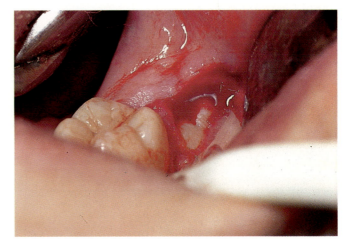

Fig. 11-32, d. Triangular flap reflected. One can see the tooth, follicle, and investing bone high on the buccal.

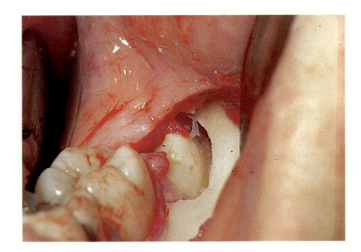

Fig. 11-32, e. Bone removal (buccal shelf, distal bone, and troughing buccally to the bifurcation).

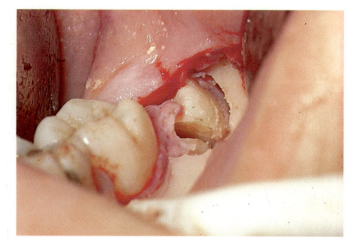

Fig. 11-32, f. Longitudinal section cut through the bifurcation, but stopping short of the lingual surface.

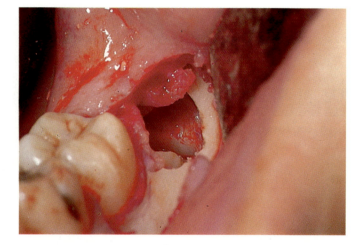

Fig. 11-32, g. Distal half removed.

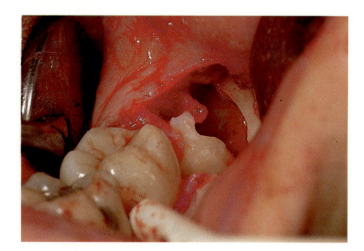

Fig. 11-32, h. Mesial half being elevated.

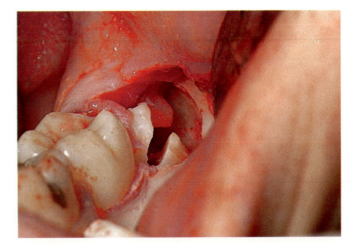

Fig. 11-32, i. Since the tooth started to bind against the second molar, it was sectioned to facilitate removal.

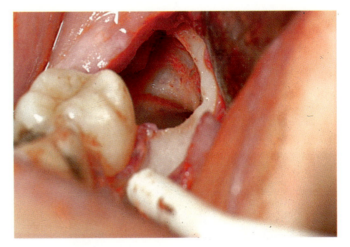

Fig. 11-32, j. Empty socket ready for follicle removal and debridement.

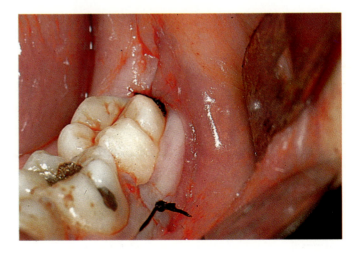

Fig. 11-32, k. Sutured case. Usually the knot is on the other side of the incision line, but this is inconsequential.

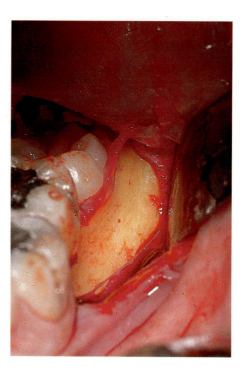

Fig. 11-33, a. Partially erupted tooth, still classified as an impaction because of high distal hard and soft tissue. Yellow bone indicates that the patient is on long-term tetracycline therapy.

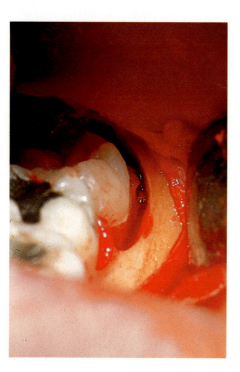

Fig. 11-33, b. Minor crestal bone removal.

Fig. 11-33, c. After elevator luxation, the tooth was removed with a forcep. Both roots fractured during the extraction, but because the tooth was sufficiently luxated and root curvatures were minimal, attached nerves were strong enough to bring the root tips out with them.

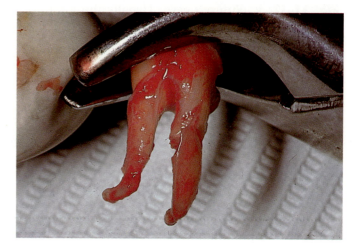

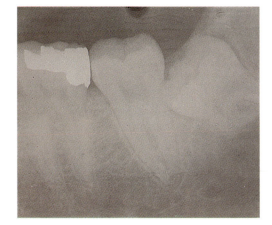

Fig. 11-34, a. Periapical x-ray of a mesioangular impaction in a 19-year-old male. Since the x-ray does not show anatomy around the apcx of the distal root, a supplemental PA or panoramic should be taken.

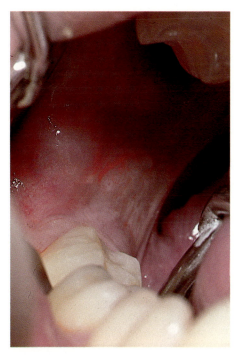

Fig. 11-34, b. Preoperative view.

Fig. 11-34, c. Flap reflected.

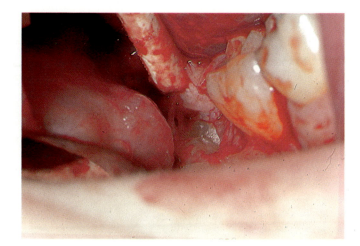

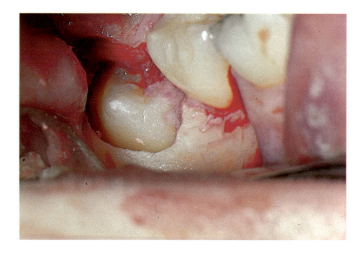

Fig. 11-34, d. Bone removal.

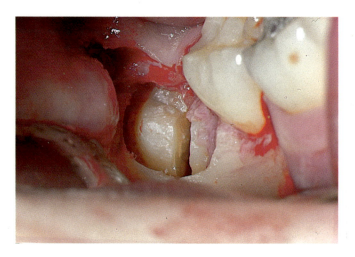

Fig. 11-34, e. Longitudinal sectioning.

Fig. 11-34, f. Distal half removed.

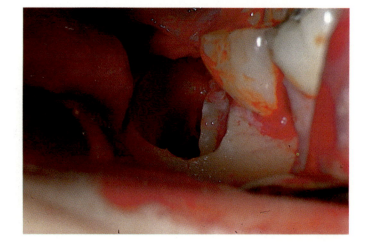

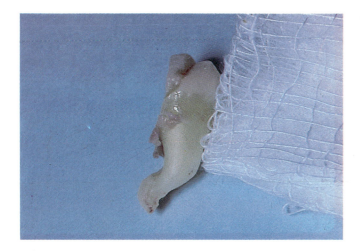

Fig. 11-34, g. Distal half of tooth.

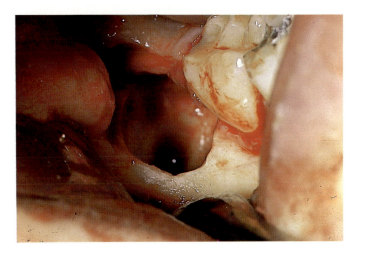

Fig. 11-34, h. Empty socket.

Fig. 11-34, i. Sutured case.

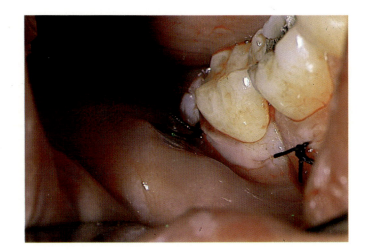

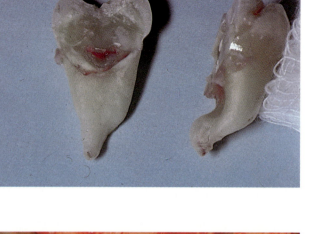

Fig. 11-34, j. Distal half of tooth on the left, mesial half on the right.

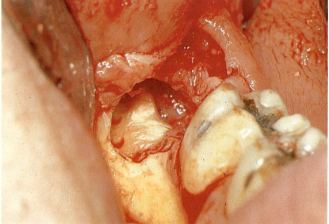

Fig. 11-35, a. Complete bony impaction. Bone has been removed to expose the crown.

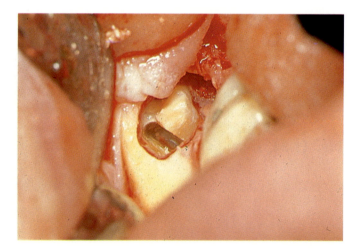

Fig. 11-35, b. The crown was removed, followed by elevation of the roots into the crown space.

Fig. 11-35, c. Empty socket.

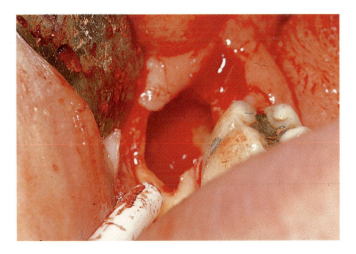

Fig. 11-35, d. Sutured case.

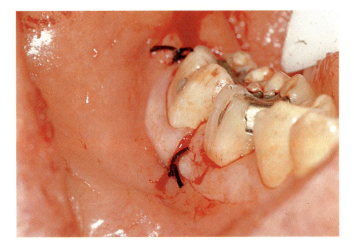

Fig. 11-36, a. X-ray of a partially erupted mandibular third molar.

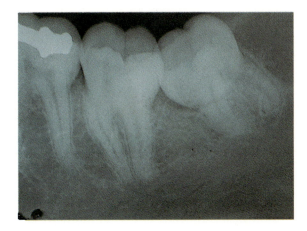

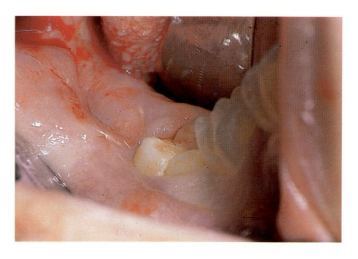

Fig. 11-36, b. An inexperienced dentist might construe this case to be easier than it actually is. Impaction removal principles are necessary to effect removal.

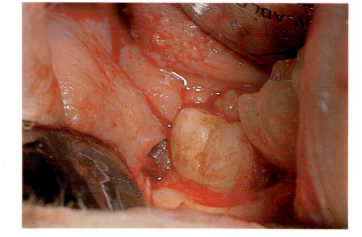

Fig. 11-36, c. As elevator and forcep implementation were to no avail, a flap was reflected for a more serious encounter with the tooth. Some distal bone was excised from over the height of contour.

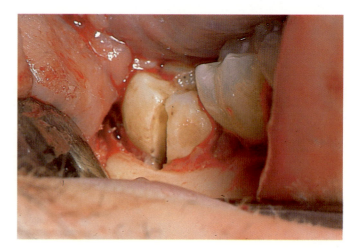

Fig. 11-36, d. Elevator and forcep use still did not bring results, so a section cut was made into the bifurcation.

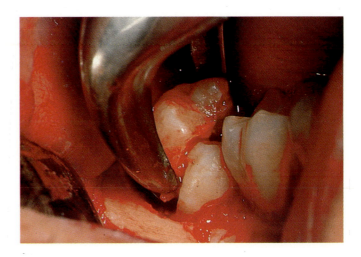

Fig. 11-36, e. Forcep removal of the distal half.

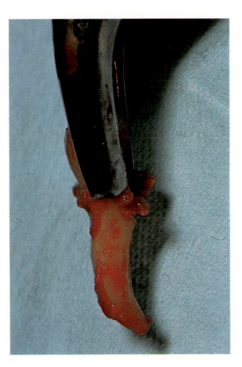

Fig. 11-36, f. Extracted segment.

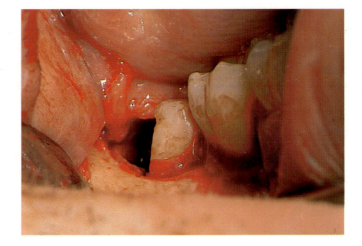

Fig. 11-36, g. A 301 elevator placed mesially allowed the coronal part of this segment to roll distally.

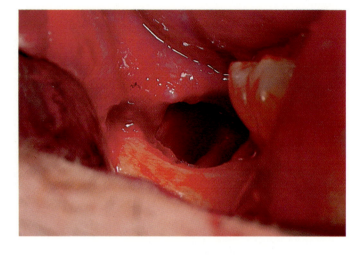

Fig. 11-36, h. Empty socket.

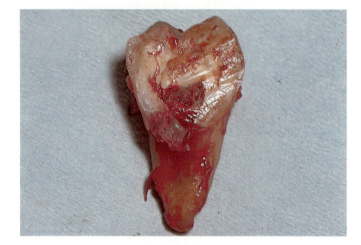

Fig. 11-36, i. Note the area of the tooth actually cut with the bur. It extends into the bifurcation but stopped short of the lingual surface of the tooth. The author recommends this procedure to protect the lingual nerve, which is generally only 2 mm below the alveolar crest and 0.5 mm from the lingual plate.

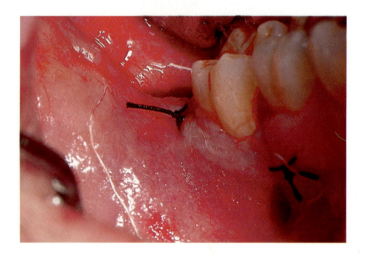

Fig. 11-36, j. Sutured case.

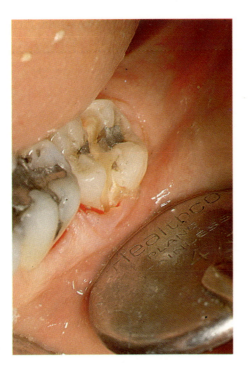

Fig. 11-37, a. Erupted third molar with curved and divergent roots. Since the tooth would not come out by only using elevators and forceps, the operator implemented the impaction technique of sectioning through the middle of the tooth, separating it into two halves. By using a forcep, the mesial half came out intact. The distal part fractured and the root was removed through the socket with a Cryer elevator.

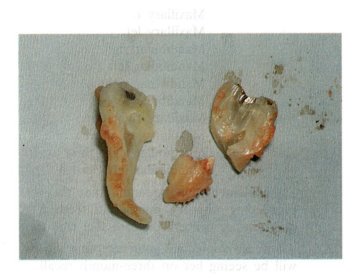

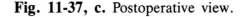

Fig. 11-37, b. Tooth fragments.

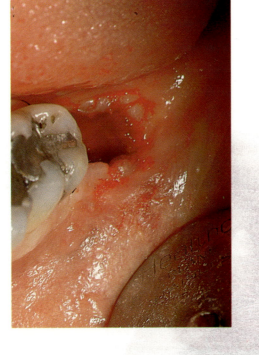

Fig. 11-37, c. Postoperative view.

Fig. 11-38, a. The orthodontist requested that 10 teeth be removed from a 12-year-old girl prior to commencing treatment:

February 12, 1985

Dr. Karl R. Koerner
19 W. Center
Logan, UT 84321

Re:

Dear Dr. Koerner:

We recently took the enclosed panoramic on a 12-year-old girl and due to the severe crowding which she exhibits, I would recommend extraction of the following teeth at this time:

Maxillary right first bicuspid
Maxillary left first bicuspid
Mandibular right first bicuspid
Mandibular left first bicuspid
Mandibular right second primary molar
Mandibular left second primary molar
Maxillary right third molar
Maxillary left third molar
Mandibular right third molar
Mandibular left third molar

I explained to her grandmother the need for these extractions and the reason for proceeding with the number of teeth recommended for extraction. If you have any questions or concerns, please feel free to call.

I would appreciate your returning the panoramic x-ray following the extractions. We will be seeing her on three-month recall.

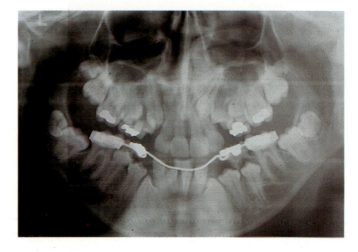

Fig. 11-38, b. Preoperative panoramic film.

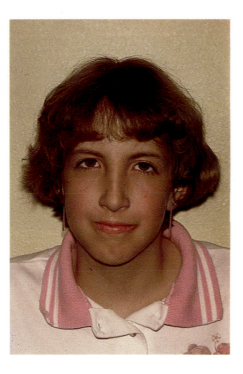

Fig. 11-38, c. This is a five-day postoperative picture of the patient. The procedure took about one hour. Oral anti-inflammatory medication greatly minimized the postsurgical morbidity.

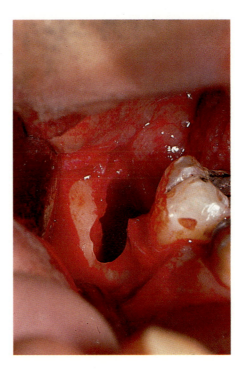

Fig. 11-39, a. This case represents an unusually large amount of bone removed for a third molar. The patient was a 35-year-old man with dense bone. Elevators and root picks were used unsuccessfully. Finally, inter-radicular bone and then more buccal bone was removed before the root was extricated. The procedure took about 20 minutes instead of the normal 5-10 minutes one might expect. Part of the problem had to do with the patient's age (see Table 11-2).

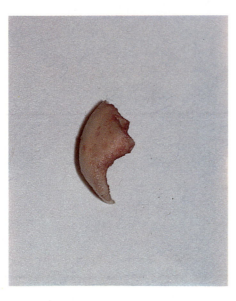

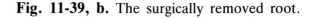

Fig. 11-39, b. The surgically removed root.

Fig. 11-40, a. High horizontal impaction.

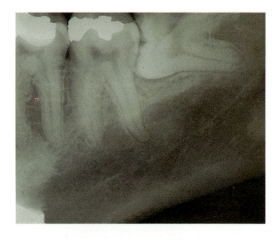

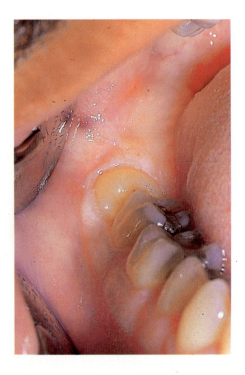

Fig. 11-40, b. Preoperative clinical view.

Fig. 11-40, c. This case exhibits some errors in judgement. Although these errors did not cause any intraoperative or postoperative problems, they could have. Three possible problems are: (1) A split-thickness rather than full-thickness mucoperiosteal flap anteriorly, (2) the distal incision being angled too far lingually, and (3) the retractor resting on the folded flap rather than bone. There were no problems with tooth or bone manipulation.

The A cut has been made from the superior cementoenamel junction inferiorly, terminating apical to the height of contour.

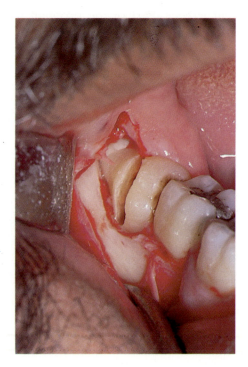

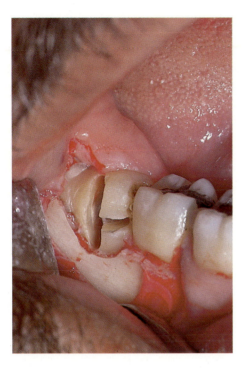

Fig. 11-40, d. Fracture of the A cut was completed with an elevator, after which the perpendicular B cut was made. This allowed removal of the crown in two parts. Some bone has been removed from the buccal. No trough was created.

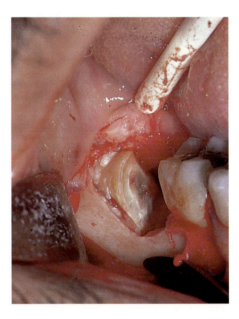

Fig. 11-40, e. With the crown gone, the root complex can be brought forward into the crown space – either intact or in two sections. Careful examination of the pulp chamber reveals the location of the root canals. This knowledge is important in deciding the angle at which to make a section cut between the roots.

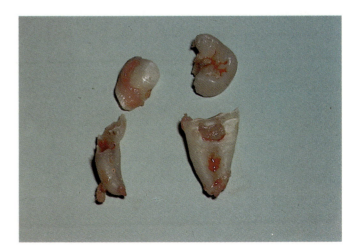

Fig. 11-40, f. Since the complete root would not slide forward, the operator performed the cut between the roots. Removing bone superiorly, exposing more root surface allows access for a purchase point and elevator (such as Crane Pick) leverage.

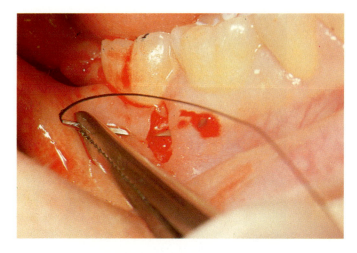

Fig. 11-41, a. One of the most difficult aspects of impaction surgery is suturing the releasing incision. A large 1/2 round needle is not suited for this task. A 3/8 circle needle shown here is more appropriate.

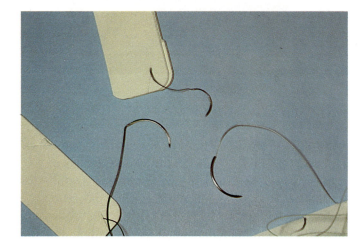

Fig. 11-41, b. This picture illustrates three types of suture material commonly used in dental offices. On the left is 4.0 silk with a 3/8 circle needle. The size of the suture material is not as important as the size of the needle. On the right is 4.0 chromic gut (resorbable in 12-14 days) with the same size needle. Above is 5.0 silk with a smaller 3/8 circle needle which is used primarily for more delicate procedures such as free gingival grafts and suturing lips.

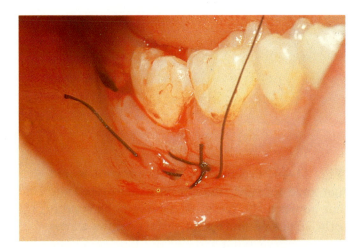

Fig. 11-41, c. Occasionally, a releasing incision will require more than one suture.

Fig. 11-42, a. Dry socket prevention. A common method of dry socket prevention includes using Gelfoam™ and either a suspension made from a tetracycline capsule or Terra-Cortril™. Predisposing factors responsible for dry sockets are smoking, birth control pills, older patients, pre-existing infection, and use of a bur deep in the socket. About one-half of a #4 Gelfoam sponge is used in each socket.

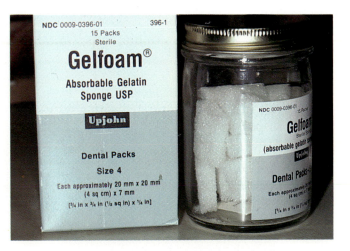

Fig. 11-42, b. Ophthalmic Terra-Cortril. The ointment form of this medication should not be used because it does not resorb.

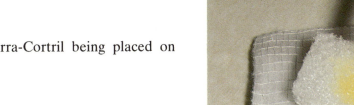

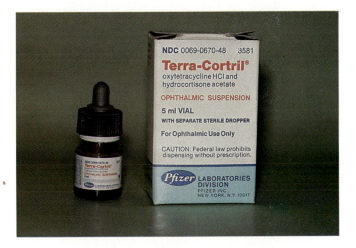

Fig. 11-42, c. Terra-Cortril being placed on Gelfoam.

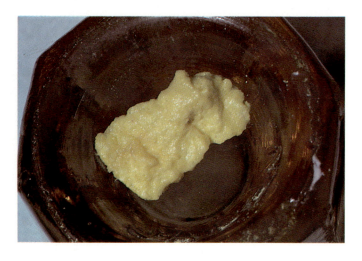

Fig. 11-42, d. Gelfoam saturated with a tetracycline suspension.

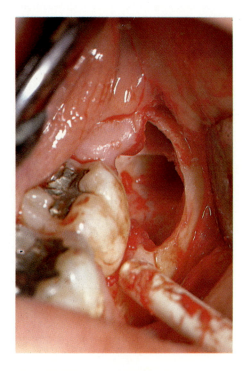

Fig. 11-42, e. Empty socket.

Fig. 11-42, f. Socket into which medication has been placed.

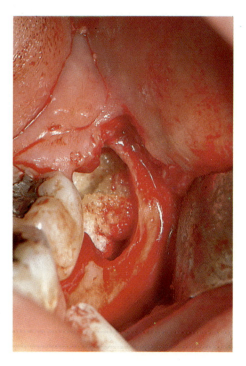

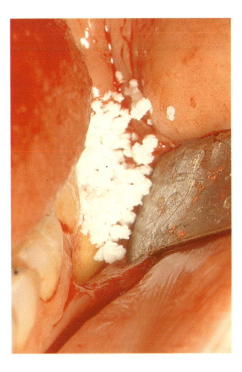

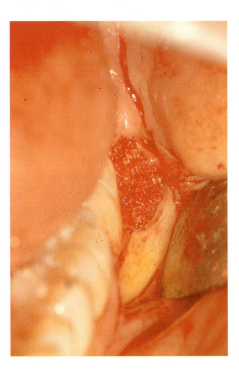

Fig. 11-42, g. This represents an alternative to medicated Gelfoam: Dry-Lac.™ It has been put in the socket with a syringe.

Fig. 11-42, h. The Dry-Lac has now been saturated with the patient's blood and the case is ready to close.

Fig. 11-43, a. Dry socket treatment. Once a dry socket is diagnosed, it is gently irrigated with warm water using an irrigation syringe, and a pack such as the one shown here is carefully placed in the socket. This packing material is iodoform gauze impregnated with a commercial dry socket paste. It is not usually necessary to anesthetize the area.

The pack is generally removed after two days, although the time period can be shorter or longer. When the pack is removed, the patient is given an irrigation syringe to use once a day as long as needed.

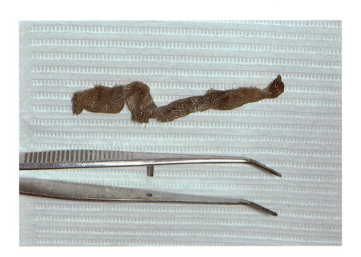

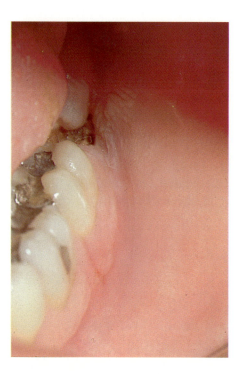

Fig. 11-43, b. Dry socket pack in place.

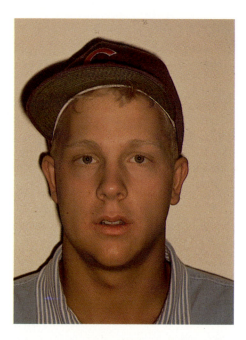

Fig. 11-44, a. Subperiosteal abscess. The patient presented about three weeks following surgery with visible facial swelling, pain, and a foul taste in the mouth. A radiograph showed nothing abnormal. Intraoral palpation over the original flap revealed swelling and tenderness and produced drainage from the distal aspect of the second molar.

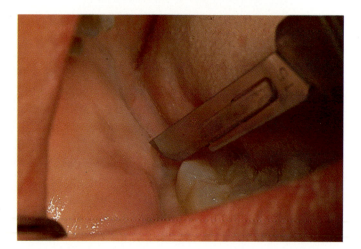

Fig. 11-44, b. The area was anesthetized and an incision was made close to the original distal incision.

Fig. 11-44, c. A purulent exudate drained spontaneously from the wound.

Fig. 11-44, d. The socket was profusely irrigated.

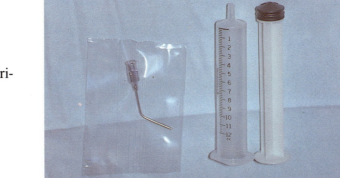

Fig. 11-44, e. It is prudent to place a drain for at least a few days to maintain patency. In this case, dry socket paste was wiped from the iodoform gauze dry socket packing material and placed into the socket.

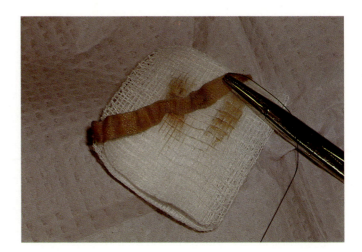

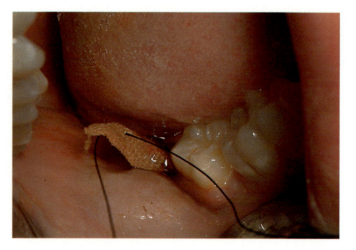

Fig. 11-44, f. The drain will be sutured in position at the incision line so that it will not fall into the socket or come out into the mouth.

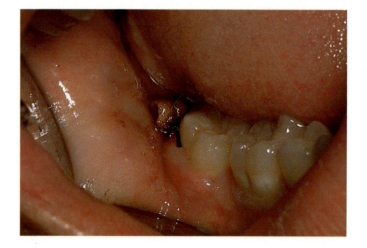

Fig. 11-44, g. Drain sutured in place. Treatment also includes an antibiotic such as Pen V K 500 mg, 2 stat and 1 qid for about one week. The drain can be removed after 2-3 days.

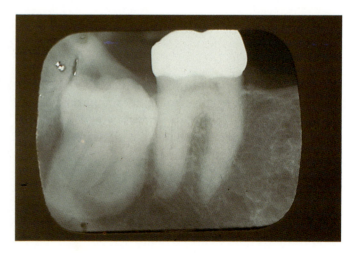

Fig. 11-45, a. If tooth removal is indicated in older individuals such as this 60-year-old man, the case should probably be referred to a specialist. Bone is dense and tightly encased around the tooth, in contrast to young patients in whom bone is quite elastic and separated from the tooth by a developmental sac and 1/4 mm periodontal ligament space.

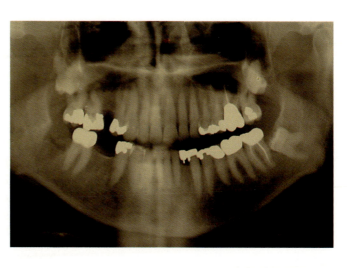

Fig. 11-45, b. Treatment of this case resulted in a fracture through the angle of the mandible.

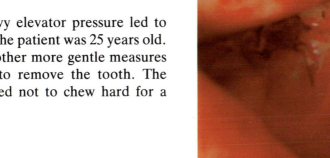

Fig. 11-45, c. Heavy elevator pressure led to this short fracture. The patient was 25 years old. Once it happened, other more gentle measures were implemented to remove the tooth. The patient was cautioned not to chew hard for a month.

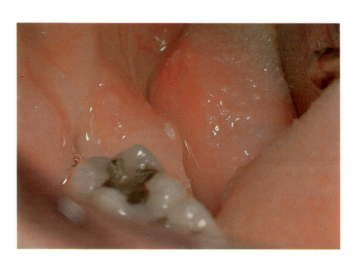

Fig. 11-45, d. This new patient presented for a consultation about two weeks after having third molars removed in another office. The lingual place was obviously expanded during the extraction. The patient was anesthetized and strong finger pressure was placed to realign the bony contour. A small piece of exposed bone was removed. There were no further problems.

Maxillary Third Molar Impactions

Surgery on maxillary third molars follows the same six steps as mandibular third molars.

Flaps

Flaps for impacted teeth will fall into one of two categories—**envelope** or **triangular**. The posterior portion is identical with either of the two. The distal-most incision point begins just anterior to the hamular notch and is then brought forward along the crest of the ridge until the blade butts against the second molar. The scalpel veers buccally into the second molar sulcus and follows the free margin anteriorly. A short envelope flap will terminate at the mesiobuccal line angle of the second molar while a longer one (for more access) will stop at the mesiobuccal line angle of the first molar. Examples of each are given in Figures 11-46, 11-47, and 11-48.

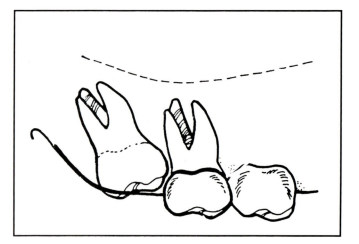

Fig. 11-46. Short envelope flap for a maxillary third molar impaction.

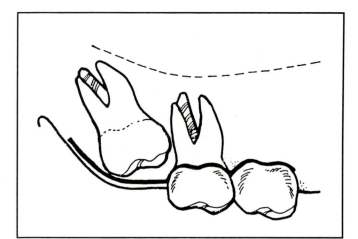

Fig. 11-47. Long envelope flap for a maxillary third molar impaction.

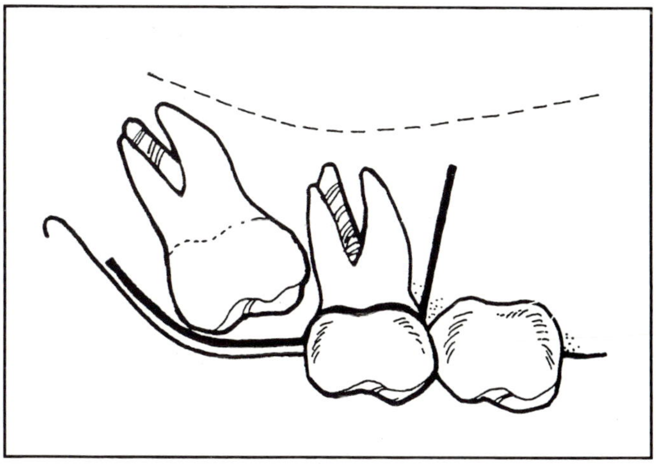

Fig. 11-48. Triangular flap for a maxillary third-molar impaction.

Bone Removal

Bone removal is predominantly from the buccal-occlusal with distal bone removal performed as needed. Buccal bone is very thin and can be excised several millimeters up the root surface if necessary to effect tooth removal.

Luxation, Sectioning, and Elevation

Since there is less cortical bone around maxillary thirds as compared to mandibular thirds, less force is required for luxation and elevation. Some operators refer to this force as "finger pressure."

Sectioning of upper third molars is the exception, not the rule. Poor visibility and inadequate access with instruments makes this a difficult job to accomplish.

Although straight elevators are commonly used for removal, difficult situations sometimes require the use of a curved elevator such as the Millers. Since the tip can be placed more to the lingual, it has the capability of exerting more of a buccal-occlusal vector of force, thus improving on the more distal-occlusal forces from straight elevators.

Avoiding Anatomic Spaces

Sometimes a maxillary third molar will inadvertently be lost into one of three anatomic spaces: the infratemporal space, the buccal or facial space, or the maxillary sinus. Three factors that will help prevent an operator from losing a tooth in one of these areas are (1) use of a triangular flap for deeper impactions, (2) use of a curved elevator, and (3) placing the periosteal elevator posterior to the tooth as it begins its descent and then letting the tooth "ride" the elevator inferiorly until it can be grasped with a forcep or hemostat.

Figure 11-49 illustrates the step-by-step approach to a moderate depth maxillary mesioangular impaction. Figures 11-50 through 11-53 present ideas to consider in removing vertical, distoangular, distohorizontal, and transverse impactions.

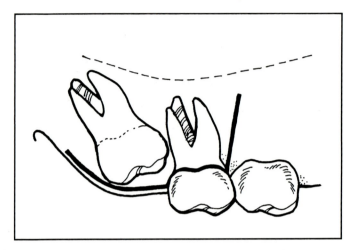

Fig. 11-49. Surgical technique for a maxillary mesioangular third molar impaction. a. Outline of the triangular flap.

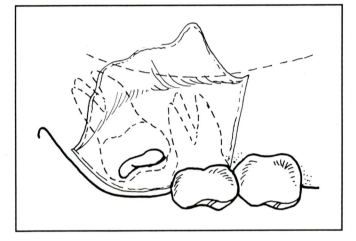

Fig. 11-49, b. Flap reflected.

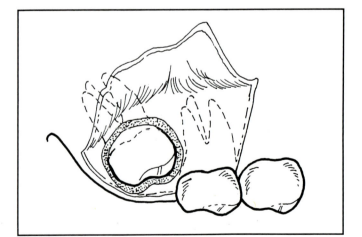

Fig. 11-49, c. Bone removal from primarily the buccal and occlusal surfaces. This bone is very thin. If necessary, bone can also be removed from the distal. It is rarely removed from the mesial except to make room to engage an elevator.

Fig. 11-49, d. A straight or curved elevator (a curved, Miller elevator is depicted in this illustration) can be applied apical to the tooth's height of contour to engage and elevate out the tooth.

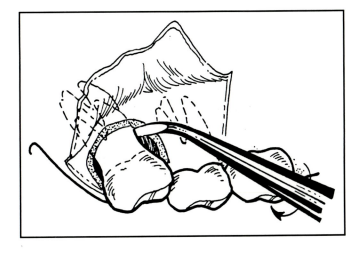

Fig. 11-49, e. Sutured case. In this drawing, one suture is shown on the buccal.

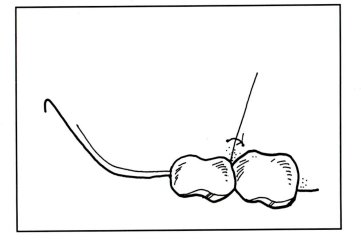

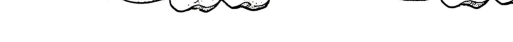

Fig. 11-50. Operative recommendations for a maxillary vertical impaction.

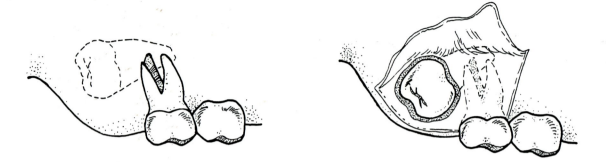

Fig. 11-51. Operative recommendations for a maxillary distoangular impaction.

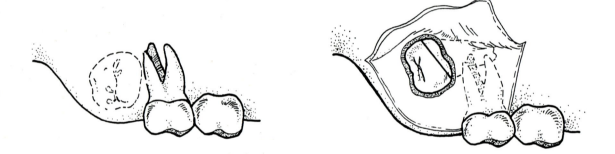

Fig. 11-52. Operative recommendations for a maxillary distohorizontal impaction.

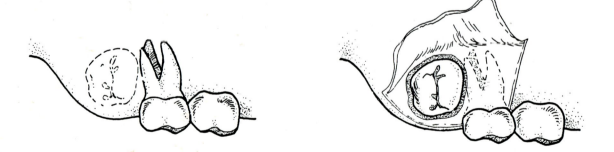

Fig. 11-53. Operative recommendations for a maxillary transverse impaction (crown to buccal).

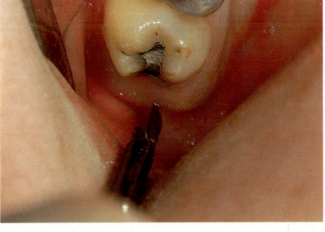

Fig. 11-54, a. The distal incision for a maxillary third molar impaction starts just anterior to the hamular notch and comes forward to the second molar along the crest of the ridge.

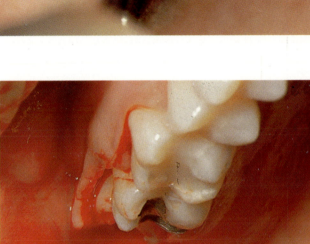

Fig. 11-54, b. Envelope flap.

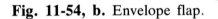

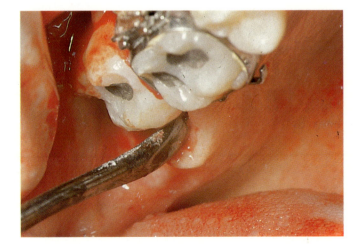

Fig. 11-54, c. Lingual gingiva often needs to be loosened so that the tooth can come down without being inhibited by fixed tissue.

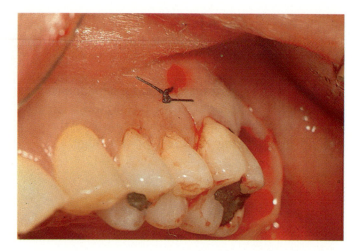

Fig. 11-54, d. Releasing incision for a triangular flap.

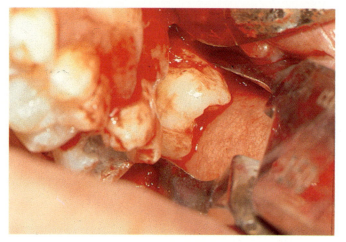

Fig. 11-54, e. In this case, a forcep is used to deliver a third molar. Due to limited access, this is not always possible.

Fig. 11-55, a. Radiograph of a maxillary partial bony impaction.

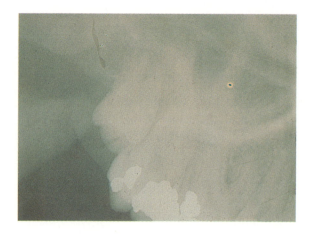

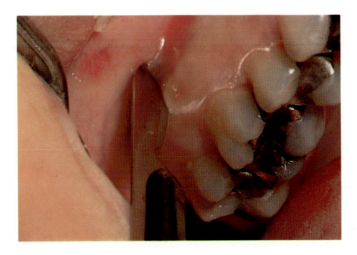

Fig. 11-55, b. Releasing incision.

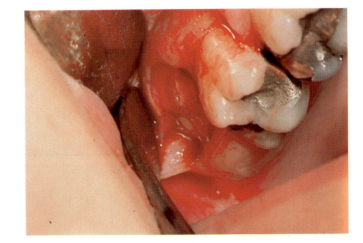

Fig. 11-55, c. Distal incision.

Fig. 11-55, d. Reflected flap—no bone removal.

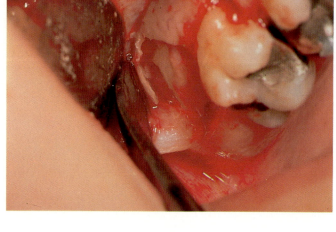

Fig. 11-55, e. Since the tooth would not come with just attempted elevation, some buccal bone was removed.

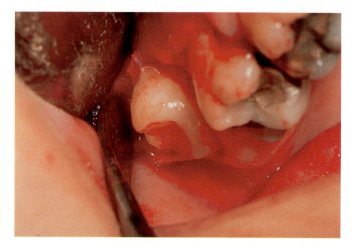

Fig. 11-55, f. The tooth then came down quite easily.

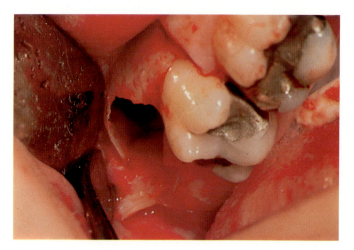

Fig. 11-55, g. Empty socket.

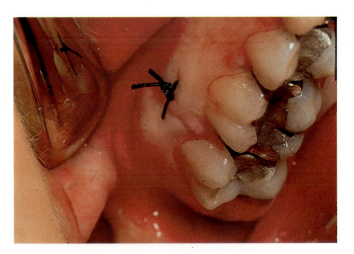

Fig. 11-55, h. Sutured case. Only one suture was placed. This operator does not use distal sutures unless there is a tissue height discrepancy between buccal and lingual greater than 1-2 mm.

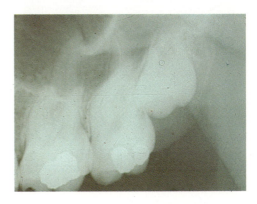

Fig. 11-56, a. Radiograph of a complete bony impaction.

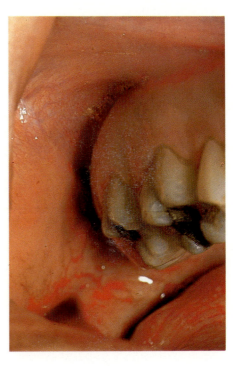

Fig. 11-56, b. Preoperative clinical view.

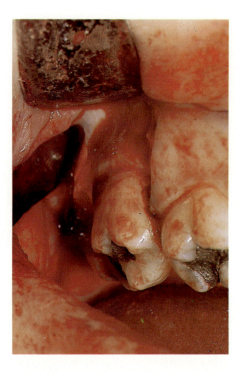

Fig. 11-56, c. Flap being reflected.

Fig. 11-56, d. The flap has been reflected and buccal and occlusal bone has been removed with the bur. Elevator placement is next.

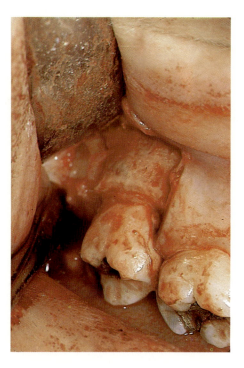

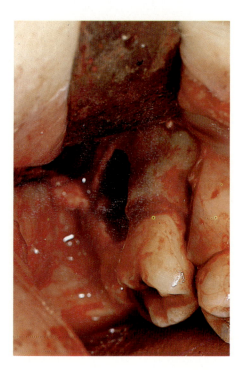

Fig. 11-56, e. Empty socket. Note the thinness of bone on the lateral surface of the alveolar process.

Fig. 11-56, f. Extracted tooth.

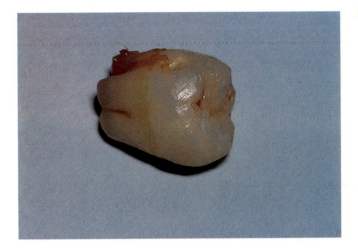

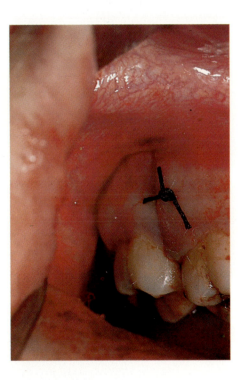

Fig. 11-56, g. Sutured case.

Fig. 11-57, a. This is the palatal surface and these are palatal roots of a maxillary, partial bony impaction. The reader can understand why normal elevator pressure with conservative bone removal failed to deliver this tooth.

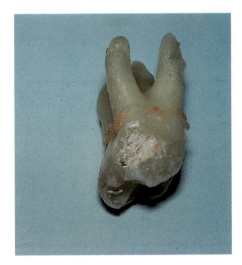

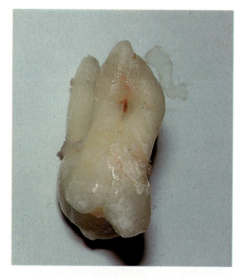

Fig. 11-57, b. Buccal surface of the tooth. Bone was removed nearly to within 3-4 mm of the apex before the tooth could be dislodged.

Fig. 11-58, a. Radiograph showing a third molar and supernumerary. *Case courtesy of Dr. Mark Phipps.*

Fig. 11-58, b. Flap reflection.

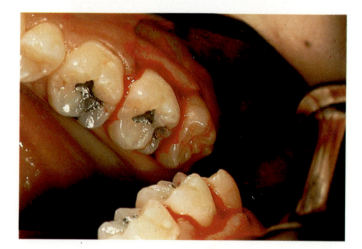

Fig. 11-58, c. The third molar has been removed.

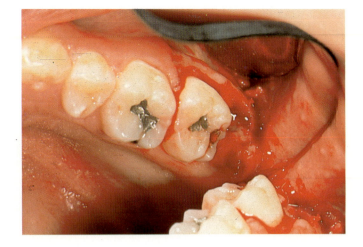

Fig. 11-58, d. The supernumerary is emerging from its deep alveolus with simple elevation. Access is through the third molar socket.

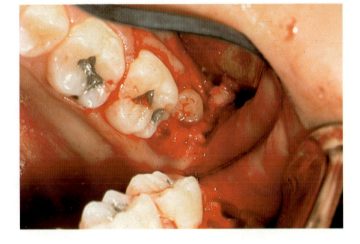

Fig. 11-58, e. Removal of the tooth from the mouth.

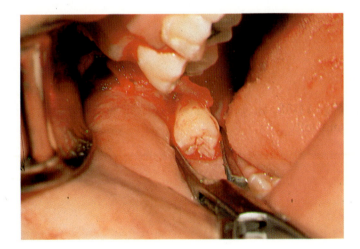

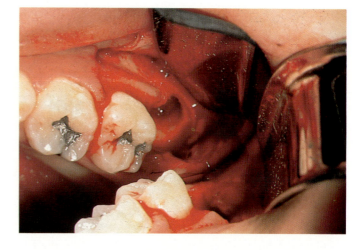

Fig. 11-58, f. Empty socket.

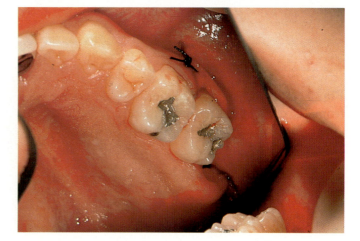

Fig. 11-58, g. Sutured case.

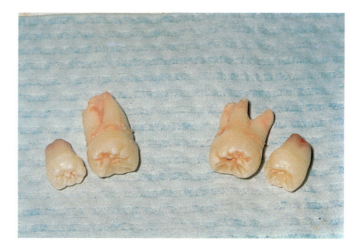

Fig. 11-58, h. Teeth removed from both right and left.

Fig. 11-59, a. This tooth was removed from a 21-year-old female without much difficulty.

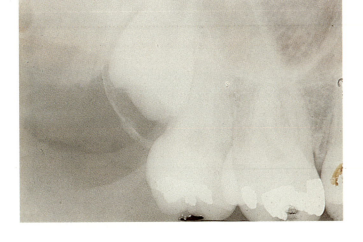

Fig. 11-59, b. Before attempting the other side (shown here), the operator first questioned the advisability of removing the tooth. The patient was comfortably sedated with oral medication. With some reservation, the doctor went ahead with the case.

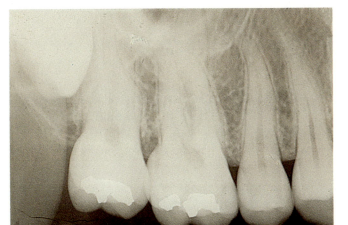

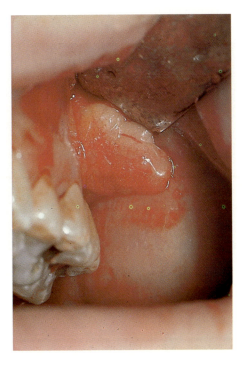

Fig. 11-59, c. A few minutes into the procedure, fat from the cheek entered the surgical field. The operator had reflected the flap higher than the mucobuccal fold (buccinator muscle attachment). At that level, facial space contents are on the opposite side of the flap. A tear in the flap allows access to loose tissue from that space, as seen here. Ostensibly, while removing buccal bone, the bur touched the periosteum of the flap, opening the communication. The fat could be poked back into the cheek but would only stay there if the retractor were held over the opening. With the fat held out of the way, the tooth was sectioned in half and removed. It was too bulbous to come out whole.

Fig. 11-59, d. The extracted tooth. The patient was placed on antibiotics because of the anatomic space contamination. There were no other complications.

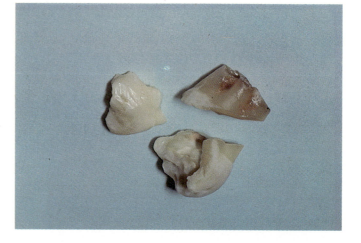

Fig. 11-60, a. Preoperatively, there was every indication that this third molar would be easy to remove.

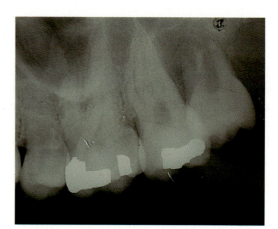

Fig. 11-60, b. During the procedure, the tooth disappeared. It was later discovered to be in the facial space, near the buccal fat pad, and it was retrieved two weeks later.

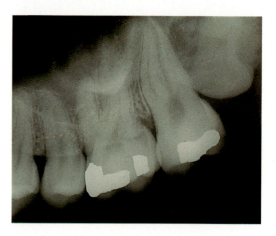

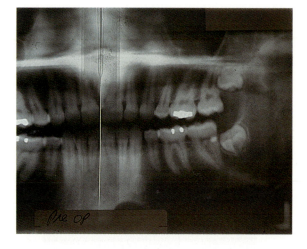

Fig. 11-60, c. This upper left impacted third molar offers a moderately difficult case.

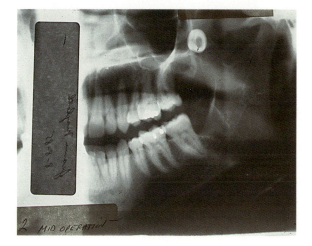

Fig. 11-60, d. During surgery, it was displaced into the infratemporal fossa. It was retrieved three weeks following the initial surgery.

In order to prevent these occurrences: (1) use a flap design that provides adequate access and visibility, then keep your eyes on the tooth as it starts to move; (2) use curved elevators, especially for more difficult cases, in order to obtain the "buccal vector of force" that comes from placing the instrument on the lingual; and (3) let the tooth "ride" an instrument (such as the periosteal elevator) out of the socket.

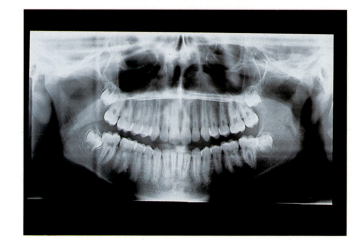

Fig. 11-6, a. Panoramic x-ray of a case involving third molars on a sixteen-year-old male. The orthodontist has requested their removal.

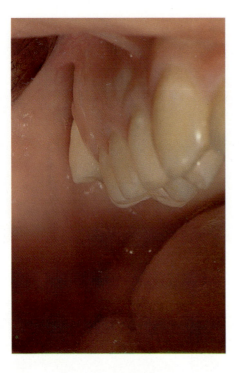

Fig. 11-61, b. Note the maxillary second molars in buccal-version—making surgical access to impacted third molars very difficult.

Fig. 11-61, c. With a releasing incision and buccal bone removal to gain needed access, the tooth was removed using a Miller elevator. The elevator's fulcrum turned out to be thin bone over the second molar's distobuccal root. During luxation and elevation, a snap was heard. After the third molar was out, the operator looked for and found the fractured distobuccal root. The patient was informed, but the situation was down played in terms of seriousness and the position of the second molar root fracture was noted. An endodontist was consulted and it was decided to follow the case, not performing further treatment at this time. Shown here: third molar and second molar distobuccal root.

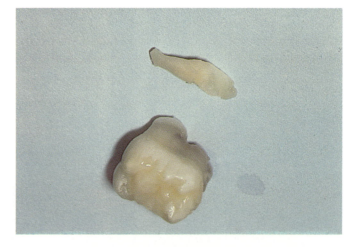

Fig. 11-61, d. X-ray taken six months postoperatively. At three years postoperatively there still were no symptoms or apparent pathology. Endodontics may ultimately be necessary.

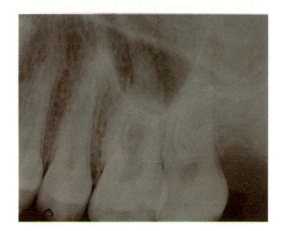

Table 11-9. Third-Molar Surgery Flowchart

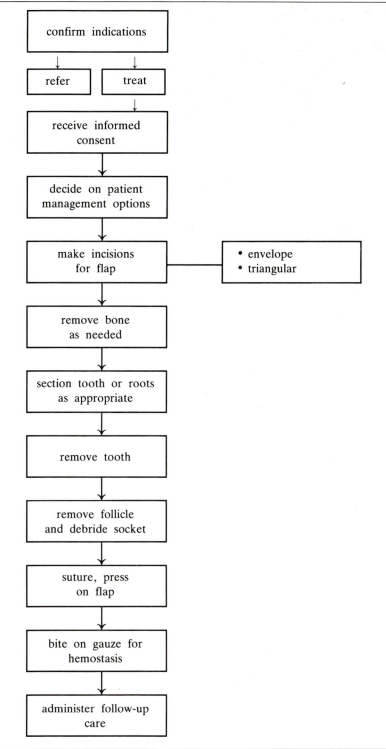

References

1. Ricketts RM. Studies leading to the practice of abortion of lower third molars. *Dent Clin North Am.* 1979;23:393.

2. Mozsary PG, and Middleton RA. Microsurgical reconstruction of the lingual nerve. *J Oral Maxillofac Surg.* 1984;42:415.

3. Bruce RA, Frederickson GC, and Small GS. Age of patients and morbidity associated with mandibular third molar surgery. *JADA.* 1980;101:240.

4. Kiesselback JE, and Chamberlain JG. Clinical and anatomic observations on the relationship of the lingual nerve to the mandibular third molar region. *J Oral Maxillofac Surg.* 1984;41:565.

Additional Reading Material

1. Koerner KR. *Clinical Procedures for Third Molar Surgery.* Tulsa, OK: PennWell Books; 1986.

2. U.S. Public Health Service, NIH. Consensus development conference for removal of third molars. *J Oral Surg.* 1980;38:235.